Svante Horsch · Luc Claeys
Editors

Spinal Cord Stimulation

An Innovative Method
in the Treatment of PVD

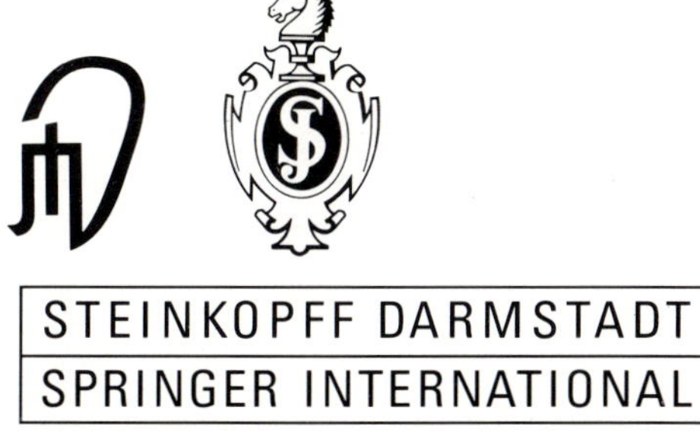

STEINKOPFF DARMSTADT
SPRINGER INTERNATIONAL

The Editors:
Prof. Dr. Svante Horsch
Dr. Luc Claeys
Krankenhaus Porz am Rhein
Akademisches Lehrkrankenhaus der
Universität zu Köln
Abteilung für Allgemeinchirurgie –
Gefäßchirurgie und Traumatologie
Urbacher Weg 19
51149 Köln

Die Deutsche Bibliothek – CIP-Einheitsaufnahme

Spinal cord stimulation: an innovative method in the treatment
of PVD / Svante Horsch; Luc Claeys (Hrsg.). – Darmstadt:
Steinkopff; Berlin; Heidelberg; New York; London; Paris;
Tokyo; Hong Kong; Barcelona; Budapest: Springer, 1994
   ISBN 3-7985-0967-0 (Steinkopff)
   ISBN 0-387-91463-3 (Springer)
NE: Horsch, Svante [Hrsg.]

Copyright © 1994 by Dr. Dietrich Steinkopff Verlag GmbH & Co. KG, Darmstadt
Medical Editor: Jens Fabry – English Editor: James C. Willis – Production: Heinz J. Schäfer
Umschlaggestaltung: Erich Kirchner, Heidelberg

Printed in Germany

Typesetting: K+V Fotosatz GmbH, Beerfelden
Printing: Betz-Druck, Darmstadt
Printed on acid-free paper

Foreword

Chronic critical limb ischemia is one of the most common causes of disability and hospitalization, and is a frequent illness in the industrialized world. There have been significant achievements in diagnostic procedures as well as in the medical, invasive, and surgical treatment of chronic critical limb ischemia in recent years. Vascular reconstruction remains the treatment of choice for patients with severe peripheral arterial occlusive disease. However, once thrombosis of the bypass has occurred, secondary procedures to restore the patency are complex and associated with 3–5 patency rates of less than 50%. The ideal treatment in nonreconstructible peripheral arterial occlusive disease should allow the patient to retain his limb with no or minimal pain and to maintain a satisfactory level of independence.

Spinal cord stimulation was introduced two decades ago by Sheally and Mortimer for the treatment of intractable pain. It gained increased interest and has subsequently been used in various fields of application. Cook, 1973, noticed an improvement in lower limb blood flow in patients who were being treated with SCS for symptoms related to multiple sclerosis. In the following years, several investigators noted pain relief and healing of ischemic ulcers in endstage vascular patients treated with SCS.

Consequently, considerable research effort was devoted to explaining the effects of SCS on pain and peripheral blood flow.

However, the selection of patients for this therapy was still largely empirical. On the other hand, the recent advances in research of the microcirculation emphasize the extremely complex pathophysiology of chronic critical limb ischemia and offers us, probably, the possibility to divide the patients into responders and nonresponders.

We are very grateful that expert clinical and experimental colleagues from around the world have joined us in the effort to provide a comprehensive book on the pathophysiology of pain and vascular pain, on the physiology behind spinal cord stimulation, on the pathophysiology of chronic critical limb ischemia and the clinical results of this innovative therapy.

This book is aimed at informing vascular surgeons and angiologists involved experimentally or clinically in studies with nonreconstructible vascular patients. The more sophisticated a method, the higher the individual expectations. However, every new method for the treatment of disabling disease has to be evaluated carefully. To encourage rational development and further discussion, insight into the individual method has to be broadened and the current "state of the art" has to be defined.

Cologne, March 1994 The Editors

Welcoming Address

On behalf of the German Society for Surgery and the German Society for Vascular Surgery, it is an honor and a pleasure for me to welcome you in Cologne to participate in this symposium on spinal cord stimulation and its therapeutic value in peripheral arterial occlusion disease. This treatment is certainly innovative, and like each new procedure, this also poses some fundamental problems.

In about 1910, in Breslau (now Wroclaw), Poland, a young surgical assistant to the famous Professor Mikulicz-Radetzki suggested to his chief the proposal to perform open-chest surgery, in the pleural lower pressure area which seemed to exclude any surgical access. Mikulicz-Radetzki answered, "With this method you could appear as a sensation in a circus." Afterwards, however, he recognized the importance of his assistant's proposal.

Another scenario: in 1929, a young surgical assisant read a paper at the annual congress of the German Society for Surgery and reported on self-experiments in catheterization of the right chamber of the heart. The chairman of this session blocked any discussion about this paper with similar words; he advised the speaker to appear as a circus attraction, and added that such experiments could certainly never be of any value for clinical medicine.

The irony of these two stories is that, first, Ferdinand Sauerbruch, one of the famous German surgeons of this century, who had invented the low-pressure chamber which enabled him to open the chest and operate on chest diseases, became the father of thoracic surgery.

Secondly, Werner Forssmann who had described his experiments on himself, introducing new diagnostic and therapeutic possibilities in cardiology and cardio-surgery, received the Nobel prize for Medicine in 1956. The moderator at the congress of the German Society of Surgery in 1929 was Ferdinand Sauerbruch. He gave Forssmann a real dressing-down, even though he himself had suffered a similar fate 20 years earlier.

The moral of these stories should be that even experts, or those who consider themselves to be experts, can be blind with regard to progressive development, especially in their speciality, and can therefore hinder scientific progress.

In the present day, endoscopic surgery is challenging the operating rooms of the world. One of its initiators was Kurt Sem, a gynecologist in Kiel, Germany, who was first humored and then attacked by prominent surgeons who called him a stubborn outsider. That was 10 years ago, and his perseverance has made it possible for this operative technique to succeed. This is yet another example of the difficulties facing innovative developments.

Let's return to electrical spinal cord stimulation. This method, a progeny of pacemaking in cardiac rhythm disorders, is certainly an innovative procedure and obviously faces the inherent problems of acknowledgment and acceptance. At present, we still have to answer a few questions: Do patients enjoy a real and lasting benefit from this treatment, and if yes, how, and to what extent? What is the cost-benefit relation? Have all these correlations been thoroughly examined?

Spinal cord stimulation presents a modern challenge in the treatment of peripheral arterial occlusive disease: it is a genuinely innovative procedure with a range of acceptance between enthusiastic encouragement and perfidious criticism.

Perhaps spinal cord stimulation has a tremendous future if it further develops to become a standard treatment in special indications. Let us try to determine if this will become reality. Our credo in innovational methods – should be to judge and measure the value of this new and, so far, unconventional therapeutic concept, not just with statistically highly significant findings, but also with patient satisfaction.

Thus, the "old" German Society for Surgery and the "young" German Society for Vascular Surgery is meeting here in historic Cologne, to set new standards, present interesting lectures and discussions, to cite further progress in our therapeutic efforts, to enrich the palette of treatment procedures, and to elucidate positive results concerning value and effectiveness of this most interesting new way of treating peripheral arterial occlusive disease.

Thank you very much for your kind attention!

Prof. Dr. med. H.-M. Becker
President of the German Society of Surgery
Chief of Vascular Surgery
Academic Teaching Hospital Munich-Neuperlach
of the University Munich
Oskar-Maria-Graf Ring 61
D-81737 Munich
FRG

Contents

Anatomy, physiology and pharmacology of pain

Basic neurophysiological mechanisms
of pain and pain control

M. Zimmermann

II. Physiologisches Institut der Universität Heidelberg, FRG

Introduction

In this article, I will give an overview of the physiological and pathophysiological mechanisms in the nervous system that are relevant for pain, with emphasis on ischemia-related pain. First of all, it is practical to subdivide pain according to the supposed pathogenic mechanisms into the following four major classes, as seen from a neurophysiologist's point of view:

- Nociceptor pain, due to excitation of high threshold sensory nerve endings by potentially destructive mechanical, thermal or chemical stimuli, or by ischemia.
- Neuropathic pain or neuralgia, due to mechanical or metabolic injury of nerves, including nerve ischemia, resulting in ectopic impulse generation in peripheral or central neurons and axons.
- Dysregulation or reactive pain, due to inadequate regulatory effects by motor, sympathetic or neurohumoral systems, e.g., pain related to muscle spasms, headache of vascular origin or ischemia pain.
- Psychosomatic pain, due to, for example, emotional stress from the social environment.

Typically, more than one of these mechanisms contribute to the chronic pain of a patient. Nevertheless, this simple classification helps to set up directions for the therapeutic strategy.

Nociceptor pain

This type of pain originates from the excitation of nociceptors in the peripheral nervous system. Nociceptor function subserves a protective system of great value for survival. Functionally identifiable nociceptors have been most extensively investigated in the skin (Fig. 1) of both man and animals [48], muscle [53], joints [64] and visceral organs [11].

In a cutaneous nerve far more than 50% of the sensory fibers have nociceptive functions. They have been found among the $A\delta$-fibers (myelinated) and the C-fibers (non-myelinated). The C-fiber group includes the efferent fibers of the sympathetic nervous system, conveying information from the spinal cord to the sympathetic effector targets in the periphery. The sympathetic fibers may also be essentially involved in the mechanisms of chronic pain (see contribution by Jänig).

The functional properties of nociceptors are summarized in Fig. 1. Strong mechanical, thermal and/or chemical stimuli elicit afferent nerve impulses in the nociceptor. The micro-environment of the nociceptor, consisting of smooth muscle,

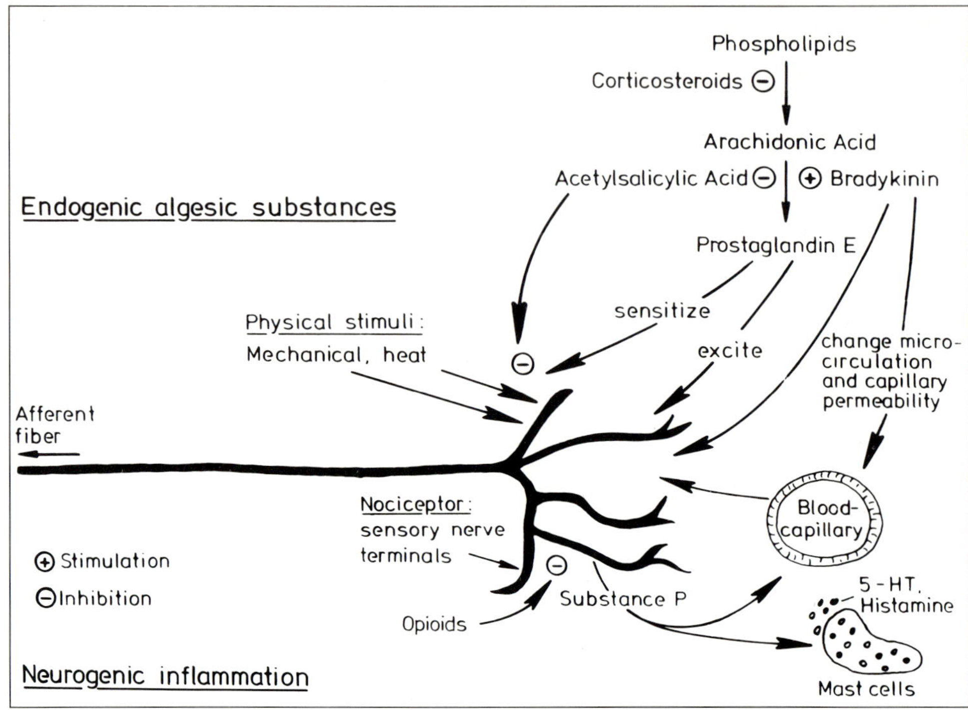

Fig. 1. The nociceptor and its micro-environment. Histologically, the nociceptor is seen as the arbor of free nerve terminals of afferent A-delta- or C-fibers. This sensory nerve ending may respond to high intensity physical stimuli and many kinds of algesic chemical substances which occur endogenously, e.g., during inflammation. In addition, the endogenous algesic substances may result in sensitization of the nociceptor. The algesic substances are vasoactive, affecting local microcirculation and increasing permeability of blood capillaries. Substance P, a neuropeptide synthesized in the spinal ganglion neurons and distributed to all parts of the primary neuron via axonal transport, is released from the nerve ending and mediates neurogenic inflammation by a direct vascular effect and by mast cell degranulation. Acetylsalicylic acid and related analgesic drugs interfere with the synthesis of prostaglandins and directly with the excitation of the nociceptor terminal. Opioids interfere with the release of substance P and may suppress the excitation of the nociceptor

blood capillaries, efferent sympathetic nerve fibers and a complex biochemical compartment, can undergo slow and lasting pathophysiological changes such as occur during inflammation. These may result in sensitization of nociceptors [62]. The pathogenic conditions and the possibilities for therapeutic interventions at the periphery, although basically established, have so far not been studied in detail.

Nociceptors have been quantitatively characterized in man and animals with experimental stimuli known to elicit painful sensations, such as controlled heating of the skin [3]. An important finding was that the discharge frequency in nociceptive afferent fibers increased with increasing skin temperature during noxious thermal stimulation (Fig. 1). Thus, nociceptors provide information on the stimulus intensity which is conveyed to the CNS by their firing rate (intensity coding).

4

Endogenous pain mediators

Endogenously occurring chemical substances (pain mediators) such as H^+-ions, serotonin, histamine, bradykinin, prostaglandins, and cytokines have excitatory effects on nociceptors, and various combinations of these substances play a causal role in the long lasting or chronic pain due to trauma, inflammation, and chronic ischemia [62].

Nociceptors can be excited to afferent discharges by the actions of these algesic substances [40, 48, 64]. At the same time, nociceptors are sensitized towards other kinds of stimuli which can explain the hyperalgesia and hyperpathia often observed in patients with inflammatory diseases. The actions of algesic substances on nociceptors show a complex synergy and mutual facilitation. For instance, the responsiveness of muscle nociceptors to bradykinin is much increased if, at the same time, serotonin or prostglandin E2 is present [53]. Since several of the algesic substances usually are simultaneously present in pathophysiologic conditions, these facilitatory interactions might be relevant for some kinds of chronic pain, including pain due to limb ischemia.

In addition to their direct excitatory effects onto the nociceptors, the algesic substances have indirect excitatory actions via their influences on the vascular system, because most of these substances are also vasoactive. One of these presumed indirect effects is the inadequate local microcirculation due to either excessive vasodilatation or vasoconstriction, depending on which kind of vasoactive substance predominates. In addition, capillary permeability is often increased by the algesic substances, resulting in extravasation of additional neuro- and vasoactive material, such as the plasma kinins or serotonin released from platelets upon trauma. Thus, the effects of these vasoactive factors might result in a disturbed physiological and chemical micro-environment of the nociceptor, which in turn may further enhance nociceptor excitability.

A most important finding was that many "sleeping" nociceptors normally exist which are not excited by noxious stimuli [49]. After an experimental inflammation had been induced, many of these sleeping nociceptors were recruited to respond to noxious or non-noxious stimuli.

Many substances such as acetylsalicylic acid interfere with nociceptor excitation and sensitization. This is a mechanism of peripheral analgesic drug action. Recent evidence suggests that opiates may also suppress inflammatory processes and nociceptor excitation, thus suggesting a peripheral site of opioid analgesic action (Fig. 1) in addition to their central effects [31]. Clinical tests have now been performed with a topical administration of opioids at an inflamed joint, and a clear analgesic effect could be shown [68].

Neurogenic mechanisms of chronic inflammation and pain

Although nervous system function normally is aimed at decreasing the effects of noxious stimulations (a mechanism generally designated as negative feedback in terms of control theory), we know of some efferent mechanisms and reactions which can contribute to the maintenance and upregulation of inflammation and pain (i.e., positive feedback). The following sections will introduce two potential cases of dysregulations of neurovascular function that may result in chronic pain and/or inflammation: dysregulations of vasodilatatory sensory neuropeptides and of the sympathetic nervous system.

Neurogenic inflammation by sensory neuropeptides

C-fibers in a somatosensory nerve possess a neurosecretory function [12], which is additional to their afferent nociceptive mechanisms. Substance P, a neuropeptide of the tachykinin group, is released from the peripheral endings of nociceptive C-fibers in the skin (Fig. 1), producing a strong local vasodilatation and plasma extravasation, with ensuing edema. Any orthodromic or antidromic excitation of C-fibers may result in the release of substance P. Other neuropeptides, e.g., calcitonin-gene related peptide (CGRP) and additional substances such as nitric oxide (NO) released from afferent nerve endings also contribute to this antidromic vasodilation.

These sensory neuropeptides stimulate mast cells and other cells of the local non-specific immune system, which in turn results in a release of vasoactive amines such as serotonin and histamine. These phenomena have been termed neurogenic inflammation. The fast spreading inflammatory response (within minutes) around a skin trauma is a well known case of neurogenic inflammation mediated by neuropeptide release from the axon collaterals of the afferent nociceptive C-fibers, a mechanism termed to axon reflex when it was discovered more than 50 years ago [45].

Experimental and clinical findings suggest that release of neuropeptides from the peripheral endings of afferent C-fibers are involved in multiple physiological and pathophysiological processes, e.g., in migraine [23], asthma [1], urinary tract inflammation [50] and inflammatory joint disease [44]. The pathophysiological mechanisms involve an increased synthesis of the neuropeptides in the dorsal root ganglion neurons and an enhanced release from their peripheral endings. Continuous release of substance P can activate inflammatory cells. For example, synoviocytes taken from arthritic patients were examined in cell culture [47]. Substance P at a concentration of 10^{-10} M resulted in the proliferation of the synoviocytes and stimulated the releases of prostaglandin E_2 and collagenase from these cells. Interestingly, contents of some neuropeptides in the synovial fluid of patients with joint disease is much different from that seen in normal subjects [41].

Release of substance P from afferent neurons can also be induced chemically by topical administration of capsaicin, a substance contained in red pepper which is known to produce the burning sensation, numbness, and decreased sensitivity of taste receptors upon administration of pepper as a spice to the oral cavity. At increasing dosage this substance first excites C-fibers and induces neurogenic inflammation, then neuropeptides are reversibly depleted and nociceptors become desensitized, and at still higher concentrations capsaicin becomes neurotoxic and may result in irreversible degeneration of peptide containing sensory neurons. The substance is contained in Capsicum which has long been used for therapeutic purposes as a counterirritative topical drug, e.g., in low back pain. Recently, transdermal capsaicin was used to treat postherpetic neuralgia, and some remarkable success has been reported [69].

Pain due to dysfunction of the sympathetic nervous system

Defective control by the sympathetic system [7, 38] plays a part in the sympathetic algodystrophies such as causalgia, Raynaud's disease, and Sudeck's atrophy. Various

6

pathophysiological mechanisms have been suggested to explain these phenomena. Direct excitatory actions on the nociceptors can be exerted by the adrenergic transmitters released from the efferent sympathetic fibers.

In addition to these direct effects on the afferent nerves there might be indirect influences via defective sympathetic effector mechanisms on the vascular regulation, such as inappropriate vasoconstriction and increased capillary filtration. Thus, sympathetic overactivity by a dysregulation of nervous control can induce ischemia and edema, and these could at least be partial mechanisms of chronic limb ischemia and the ensuing pain.

Reflex mechanisms might further contribute to the development and maintenance of chronic sympathetic dysfunction and the related ischemia and pain states. Recent animal studies have indeed shown that peripheral trauma can result in lasting changes of motor and sympathetic reflexes. These changes indicate central nervous system plasticity in response to peripheral injury. In cases of abnormal efferent sympathetic influences on nociceptors or on microcirculation (as discussed above) these reflexes can give rise to positive feedback loops which in turn further enhance nociceptor responsiveness and result in maintained pain. In his contribution to this volume, Dr. Jänig will provide more detail on the dysregulation of the sympathetic nervous system.

It is conceivable that both a deficiency of vasodilatatory neuropeptides from afferent neurons (e.g., substance P, CGRP) and excessive release of noradrenaline and VIP from the sympathetic nerve fibers are involved in hypoperfusion and ischemia of a limb. Therefore, it must be the aim of therapeutic measures to interfere with the underlying nervous dysregulations. Whereas we understand the relief of ischemia and pain that can be obtained by repeated sympathetic blocks with a local anesthetic, the beneficial effects are less clear of electrical spinal cord stimulation.

The synthesis of some endogenous opioids and other neuropeptides in the central nervous system is also increased during experimentally induced polyarthritis and following peripheral nerve lesions [21, 37, 54]. As release of the endogenous opioids may result in pain inhibitory functions in the central nervous system, their increased synthesis suggests a regulatory response of the nervous system aimed at decreasing the central nervous sensitivity towards the chronic nociceptive sensory inflow.

Mechanisms of neuropathic pain

Nerve lesions such as nerve or root compression (e.g., in the carpal tunnel syndrome or lumbar disk herniation), as well as polyneuropathies or zoster virus infection, result in neuropathic pain. Pain etiologies and subjective descriptions by patients show that neuropathic pain is different from nociceptor pain. Neuropathic pain often is severe and does normally not respond well to analgesic drugs. Rat models of neuropathic pain have been developed, using transection, constriction or ischemia of a peripheral nerve. These animals show behavioral signs of pain that can be treated, for example, by amitryptiline [67].

The following pathophysiological mechanisms have recently been identified in animal models and clinical studies which presumably contribute to neuropathic pain:

– After prolonged compression of a nerve or spinal root nerve fibers become sensitive to slight mechanical stimulation [4, 36, 59]; their continuous abnormal excitation thus may at least contribute to chronic pain.

- Microcirculation within the peripheral nerve (via the vasa nervorum) might become impaired by a sustained nerve compression, and secondary nerve damage can result from the ensuing ischemia of the nerve [57].
- In nerve end neuroma abnormal excitatory coupling takes place between the efferent sympathetic fibers and the afferent nociceptive fibers [39].
- Axonal transport is impaired or interrupted in both directions in the nerve fibers. This interferes with orthograde transport of neurotransmitters from the cell body to the sites of release, and with retrograde transport of neurotrophic substances taken up at the nerve fibers ending, such as nerve growth factor (NGF), that control biosynthesis in the nerve cell body. For example, gene expressions of substance P and CGRP are reduced, and those of galanin and nitric oxide synthase are increased following axotomy of dorsal root ganglion neurons [24, 32]. Thus, these sensory neurons change their biochemical and functional properties after axotomy, which include abnormal impulse generation and sympathetic coupling as mentioned above.
- Biochemical and electrophysiological abnormality induced by a lesion in primary afferent neurons spreads transsynaptically to second and higher order neurons in the spinal cord and brain [18]. These central alterations include a multitude of long lasting biochemical responses in neurons and glial cells. Spinal sensory neurons tend to become hyperexcitable, lose their inhibitory controls, and change their synaptic circuitry [77].

Thus, the effects of nerve damage are not confined to the site of trauma as had been previously believed. Rather, a series of long lasting biochemical and cellular events takes place in the damaged neuron itself and in the synaptically connected spinal neurons, which result in hyperexcitability of ascending spinal neurons and of spinal sympathetic and motor reflexes. This plasticity of nervous system function can be considered a process of learning and adaptation so that neuronal pain responses are continuously generated – chronic neuropathic pain thus appears as being due to a nervous system engramme that perpetuates a response irrespective of a peripheral stimulus.

Processing of pain-related information in the central nervous system

Pain in its subjective, behavioral and physiological expressions is based on complex interactions of neuronal systems in the spinal cord, brainstem, diencephalon, limbic system, and neocortex. Best understood are the functions of the spinal cord, and therefore spinal nociceptive functions will be detailed here as examples for central nervous mechanisms of the processing and inhibition of pain related neuronal information (Fig. 2).

Spinal neurons that transmit nociceptive informations

Most of the spinal neurons that receive input from nociceptors are multireceptive, i.e., they are activated also by low threshold mechanoreceptors. They project to the brainstem and thalamus via the anterolateral spinal tract [72]. We do not yet understand the decoding principles according to which the brain extracts the pain related

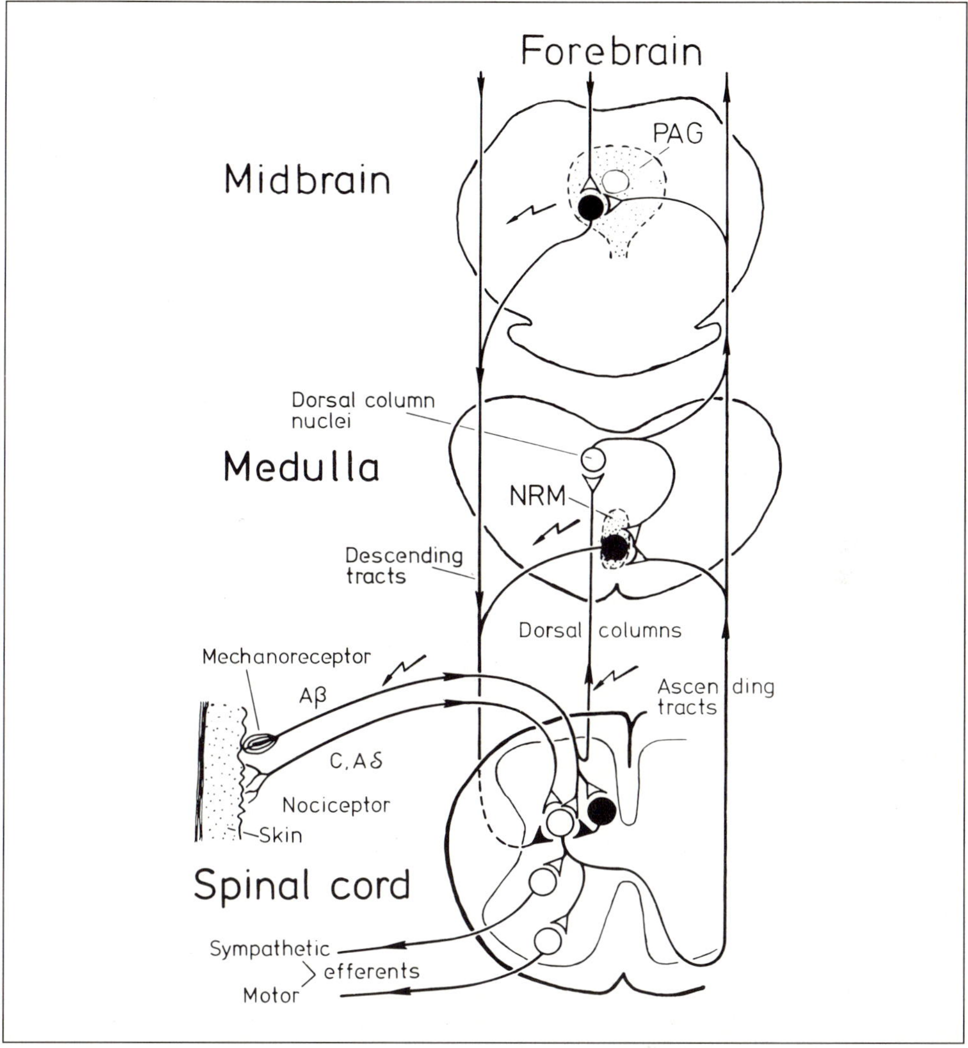

Fig. 2. Schematic diagram of the transmission and modulation of pain-related information in the spinal cord and brain, and some inhibitory nervous mechanisms involved (shown in black). Nociceptive afferent fibers (C, A delta) form excitatory synapses to dorsal horn neurons, the information of which is distributed to spinal sympathetic and skeletomotor circuits (reflexes) and ascending systems that project to various sites in medulla, mid-brain and forebrain. Both segmental spinal and descending inhibitory systems are included, if activated they modulate both the spinal reflex and ascending systems. Descending inhibition of neurons in the spinal dorsal horn can be elicited from the mid-brain (e.g., periaqueductal gray, PAG) and the medullary nucl. raphe magnus (NRM). Both these nuclei have excitatory input from the spinal cord, including the dorsal horn neurons that in turn are under descending control from PAG and NRM. The descending inhibitory systems can be activated by electrical stimulation from multiple sites (as indicated by "electrical arrows"), including the peripheral afferent nerves (transcutaneous electrical nerve stimulation, TENS) and the spinal cord (spinal cord stimulation, SCS)

information from the multireceptive neuronal discharges, although it may be somehow mediated by the pattern of a neuronal collective discharge [42, 60, 76]. However, multireceptive neurons help to understand those types of pain which are elicited or aggravated by tactile stimuli, e.g., allodynia in sympathetic reflex dystrophy to trigeminal neuralgia (tic douloureux). In these cases the ensemble of multireceptive neurons may have become abnormally excitable so that a low threshold mechanical skin stimulus triggers a brust of impulses that normally does not occur [63].

Inhibitory control of pain-related information in the central nervous system

Multireceptive neurons are subject to spinal and supraspinal inhibitory influences (Fig. 2) that play a role in the physiological control of pain sensation [2, 6, 22, 25, 71, 75]. This control of sensory functions in the spinal cord has continuous (tonic) and transient (phasic) components. The tonic inhibition has been shown in anesthetized animals by a cold block of spinal descending pathways, resulting in an increase of dorsal horn neuronal responses to noxious skin heating. On the other hand, the dorsal horn nociceptive responses can be inhibited by stimulation in the periaqueductal gray (PAG) of the midbrain or the nucleus raphe magnus (NRM) in the medulla (Fig. 2). Characteristically the inhibition upon PAG stimulation appears as a change in the slope of the encoding line relating the intensity of the heat stimulus to the response rate of the neuron. This can be interpreted as gain control of the dorsal horn neuronal system for the transmission of nociceptive information [9].

Many of the brain structures from where analgesia and descending inhibition can be induced by focal electrical stimulation are rich in opiate receptors [2]. It has been suggested therefore that the analgesic effect of opiates might be due to the activation of inhibitory systems arising from these structures, including the descending influences to the spinal cord. Indeed, injection of minor amounts of morphine at various brainstem sites elicits analgesia [74] as well as descending inhibition of dorsal horn neurons [22, 28]. However, other mechanisms exist as well that contribute to the analgesia by systemic opioids. In addition, other inhibitory neurotransmitters also play a role in pain inhibition.

A survey of the presumed excitatory and inhibitory neurotransmitters on the dorsal horn neuron is shown in Fig. 3. Synaptic transmission involves fast and slow transmitters in a synergistic and cooperative way. Usually, fast transmitters are amino acids or amines, whereas slow transmitters are neuropeptides. Substance P appears to be a major slow excitatory transmitter for pain-related information carried via impulses in nociceptive C-fibers. Putative fast neurotransmitter for nociceptive (and non-nociceptive) information are glutamate and aspartate. Many inhibitory synapses have been found to be at work on the dorsal horn neuron, some of which have been included in Fig. 3. Enkephalin and dynorphin have been localized in inhibitory spinal interneurons. The pre- or postsynaptic receptors for these endogenous opioids can be activated by spinally administered opiates, which is now a clinically most powerful procedure for analgesia.

Other segmental inhibitory mechanisms are related to gamma-aminobutyric acid (GABA); this transmitter has inhibitory functions directly on the motoneurons, as well as on the dorsal horn neurons. Baclofen, an agonist of GABA, therefore has multiple spinal sites of action, mediating the antispastic and analgesic potencies of

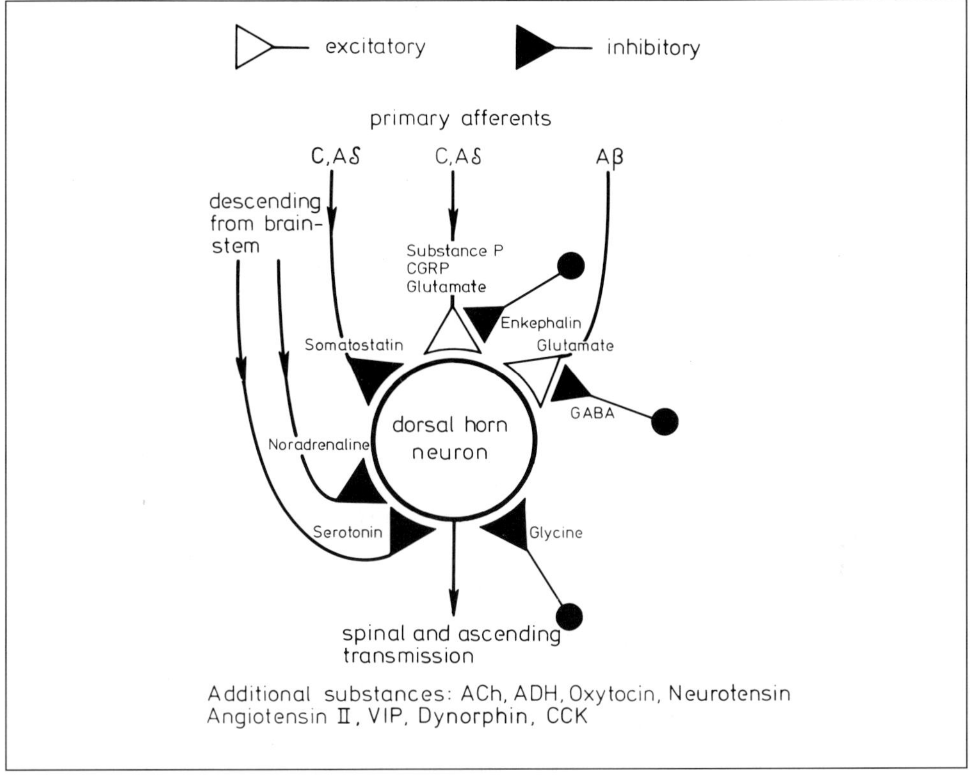

Fig. 3. Schematic diagram of the transmission of pain-related information in the spinal dorsal horn neuron, with both excitatory (shown by white synapses) and inhibitory (shown by black synapses) mechanisms involved. Both segmental spinal and descending inhibitory systems are included. Putative neurotransmitter substances are indicated. The convergence of some excitatory and inhibitory synaptic terminals onto a dorsal horn neuron is schematically shown, summarizing data from behavioral-pharmacological, neurophysiological, histochemical, and neurochemical studies. Some additional putative transmitters (not shown) have been localized histochemically in the dorsal horn, e.g., acetylcholine, neurotensin, vasoactive intestinal peptide (VIP), dynorphin, calcitonin gene-related peptide (CGRP), cholecystokinin (CCK)

this drug. Serotonin (5-HT) and noradrenaline have been identified as transmitters involved in descending inhibitory controls of nociceptive transmission in the dorsal horn.

Inhibition of central nociceptive messages by peripheral nerve or spinal cord stimulation

Inhibition of nociceptive responses of dorsal horn neurons can be performed by stimulation of peripheral nerves [14, 19, 29], which mimicks the clinical effects of TENS (transcutaneous electrical nerve stimulation). Stimulation of the dorsal columns of the spinal cord also produces inhibition of dorsal horn neurons [46], which might be the basis for pain treatment with SCS (spinal cord stimulation). Stimulation of Aβ-fibers was sufficient to elicit inhibition. However, increasing the strength of the repetitive nerve stimulus to levels recruiting Aδ and C-fibers gradually increased the inhibition which outlasted the period of stimulation. Both segmental and supraspinal inhibitory mechanisms can contribute to the observed inhibition. The supraspinal contribution was particularly significant when high-threshold afferents were recruited by the nerve stimulation, or when noxious stimuli were used to trigger the inhibition. In these cases, the inhibition could be elicited from virtually all parts of the body, suggesting the label "DNIC − diffuse noxious inhibitory control" [43]. Most likely the counter-irritation procedures known in traditional medicines all over the world, and acupuncture, also trigger the activation of endogenous inhibitory systems [70].

Recently, we have addressed the question of whether spinal inhibition induced by afferent stimulation would be enhanced by treatment of the animals with B-vitamins [26]. We found that the maximum inhibition of nociceptive transmission in lumbar spinal dorsal horn neurons of rats induced by electrical stimulation of a heterotopic limb was considerably increased by 1 week of daily applications of vitamins B_1, B_6 and B_{12}. If this additive antinociceptive effect is extrapolated to a clinical situation one may predict a facilitation of pain relief by TENS and SCS during prolonged systemic treatment with B-vitamins.

Many behavioral and neurophysiological experiments can be interpreted by assuming that, during PAG-stimulation, serotonin (5-HT) is released as an inhibitory neurotransmitter or neuromodulator from the descending neurons in the spinal cord [2]. The idea that some chronic pain may depend on a deficient central inhibitory 5-HT system has led to attempts to treat pain by dietary measures [16, 66], e.g., by supplementation of food with tryptophan, the precursor of 5-HT. Some increase of pain tolerance or decrease of chronic pain has been reported in animals and humans, and this has been attributed to increased 5-HT levels in the CNS.

Spinal cord or transcutaneous nerve stimulation can improve ischemic pain

Ischemia of a limb or the cardiac muscle usually are painful diseases that require causal and/or symptomatic treatment [51]. The experimental neurophysiological results outlined above can explain some clinical benefits of SCS and TENS in patients with painful ischemic diseases. The discharges of thoracic spinal dorsal horn neurons that receive input from cardiac afferent fibers were studied in monkeys [13]. Spinal cord stimulation inhibited the nociceptive discharges, e.g., those elicited by intracardial injection of bradykinin.

The results corroborate clinical findings in patients with pain due to an ischemic limb or cardiac ischemia. For instance, in patients with angina pectoris both the cardiac ischemia and the anginal pain were reduced by SCS [17]. In patients with severe ischemia of the lower limb 2 years of SCS treatment resulted in a considerable therapeutical improvement [27]. Laser Doppler flowmetry showed in patients with hindlimb ischemia that SCS resulted in increases of microcirculation, presumably by inhibiting steady state sympathetic excitation [55, 65]. However, this approach was not successful in diabetic patients with autonomic neuropathy.

Thus, SCS may have two inhibitory mechanisms to induce these improvements: inhibition in the central nervous system (most likely in the spinal cord) of neuronal

12

messages conveyed to the cortex or other structures that are relevant for pain sensation, and inhibition of the sympathetic vasoconstrictor neurons resulting in a relative vasodilatation of vessels suffering from occlusive pathology [65]. The latter mechanism obviously does not work in patients with an autonomic neuropathy, as in these cases the efferent sympathetic axons to the resistance vessels fail to conduct impulses, and therefore no inhibitory processes at the spinal preganglionic sympathetic neuron will become manifested at the vascular level.

Pain-induced changes of neuronal gene transcription — a pathobiological mechanism of chronic pain?

Animal experiments have revealed that long lasting modifications occur in the central nervous system in response to a noxious peripheral event [15]. For example, the threshold of the flexor reflex in rats was decreased for weeks in both hindlimbs after a transient burn trauma had been performed on one leg [73]. Experimental inflammation of a limb in rats results in upregulation of tachykinin receptor mRNA and nitric oxide (NO) synthase in the spinal dorsal horn [33], gene expression is increased of (pro)dynorphin [35, 58], and opioid receptor binding is modified [5]. These slow and long-lasting biochemical and cellular processes in the spinal cord may contribute to the hyperalgesia that outlasts the inflammation.

Nerve lesions also induce long-lasting changes in the nervous system that parallel the behavioral signs of pain and hyperalgesia [4]. For example, the patterns of sympathetic reflexes to skin and muscle were persistently changed after transection of a peripheral nerve, an observation that has been associated with sympathetic reflex dystrophy [8]. The gene expressions in spinal dorsal horn neurons of prodynorphin and dynorphin are dramatically increased after a peripheral nerve or spinal cord lesion [61]. These profound changes justify to speak of pain as a CNS disease [10].

From the available body of evidence it is conceivable that virtually and long-term change of nervous system function is preceded by modifications in gene expression in nerve cells (Fig. 4). At the DNA level processes of transcription control can be assessed by studying the immediate-early genes (IEGs) such as c-fos and c-jun, which appear to be "master switches" of the transcription machinery [30, 56]. Therefore, we have studied the induction of IEG encoded proteins in the somatosensory system under various noxious conditions.

We used immunohistochemistry to detect the IEG encoded proteins such as c-Fos, Fos B, c-Jun, Jun B, Jun D, and Krox-24 in neurons of the spinal cord and dorsal root ganglia. We observed consistent induction of all of these IEGs as early as 1 h after a noxious stimulus to a limb [34], whereas non-noxious stimulation was without effect. Depending on the degree of the noxious stimulus IEG protein expression could last for several days. It is known that the IEG encoded proteins are transcription factors that induce transcription of other genes. Thus, it is conceivable that IEG induction will be followed by expression of several target genes and de novo protein synthesis, as is schematically outlined in Fig. 4.

IEG activation was much pronounced after nerve lesions. In the neuronal cell bodies of the axotomized neurons (e.g., DRG neurons after transection of the sciatic nerve), we found a selective expression of c-Jun and Jun D, but not of the many other IEGs that can be induced transynaptically. c-Jun persisted for many months and eventually was turned off when the nerve fibers had grown to an innervation ter-

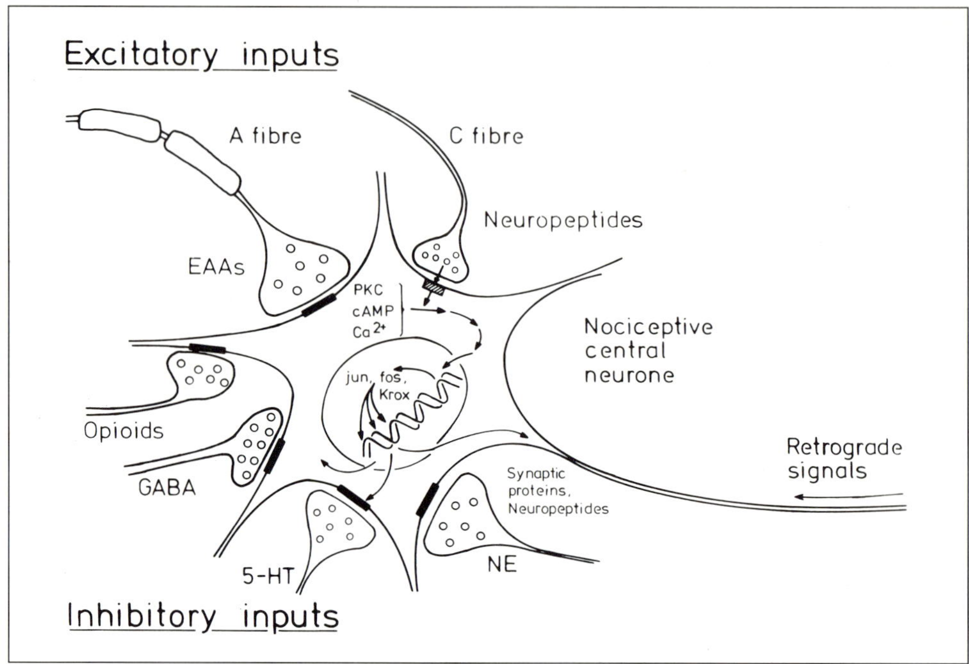

Fig. 4. Schematic diagram of stimulation-transcription coupling in nerve cells. Stimulations of a neuron by excitatory inputs can induce, via second messengers, activation of immediate-early genes (IEGs, such as fos, jun, krox-24) in the cell nucleus. The protein products of these IEGs control the expression of other genes relevant for the synthesis of constituents of neuronal function, e.g., neurotransmitters, synaptic proteins, channel proteins, enzymes. Nociceptive inputs via neuropeptides released from C-fibers, excitatory amino acids (EAAs) or signals travelling retrogradely with axonal transport can activate the transcription controlling cascade of events shown. Hypothetically, noxious stimuli and lesions of the axon can result in changes of neuronal excitability by increasing the gain of excitatory transmission, or by decreasing the efficacy of inhibitory systems. The diagram based on results and ideas by several authors as discussed in the text (from Zimmermann 1991)

ritory. After the nerve transection it took several h until c-Jun could be detected in the neuron's nucleus, depending on the distance between the site of the lesion and the cell body. With a variable delay c-Jun activation was followed by enhanced expression of the neuropeptide galanin and nitric oxide synthase [24], the enzyme responsible for the synthesis of NO, a novel neuromediator that is involved also in the transmission of noxious stimuli [52].

We hypothesize that IEG induction by noxious conditions and nerve trauma are the initial molecular steps in the development of pathophysiological properties of neurons, a most crucial one being hyperexcitability as a mechanism of chronic pain. These changes might be based upon the synthesis of inappropriate and dysfunctional neurotransmitters and synaptic receptor proteins, as indicated in Fig. 4. Thus, it is conceivable that transcription control is involved in the development of those types of chronic pain that outlast a peripheral trauma. Therefore, the investigation of neuronal IEG responses in experimental pain situations could provide access to the molecular genetic basis of chronic pain.

14

Summary and conclusions

The insights gained from basic neurobiological research have led to new ideas about the mechanisms behind hitherto unexplained phenomena of chronic pain, and have brought about considerable improvements in our concepts of pain diagnosis and therapy. On the other hand, the worldwide exchange of information and cooperation between clinical practice and basic research have been particularly fruitful in promoting pain research. The evolving concepts no longer regard pain as simply a symptom, as an indicator of pathology, but rather as an independent problem of major importance in medical thought and action.

Acknowledgements. The author's research is being supported by the Deutsche Forschungsgemeinschaft (grants Zi 110).

References

1. Barnes PJ (1992) Neural mechanisms in asthma. Br Med Bull 48:149–168
2. Basbaum AI, Fields HL (1984) Endogenous pain control systems: brainstem spinal pathways and endorphin circuitry. Ann Rev Neurosci 7:309–338
3. Beck PW, Handwerker HO, Zimmermann M (1974) Nervous outflow from the cat's foot during noxious radiant heat stimulation. Brain Res 67:373–386
4. Bennett GJ, Xie Y-K (1988) A peripheral mononeuropathy in rat that produces disorders of pain sensation like those seen in man. Pain 33:87–107
5. Besse D, Lombard MC, Besson JM (1992) Plasticity of mu and delta opioid receptors in the superficial dorsal horn of the adult rat spinal cord following dorsal rhizotomies: A quantitative autoradiographic study. Eur J Neurosci 4:954–965
6. Besson JM, Chaouch A (1987) Peripheral and spinal mechanisms of nociception. Physiol Rev 67:67–168
7. Blumberg H (1988) Zur Entstehung und Therapie des Schmerzsyndroms bei der sympathischen Reflexdystrophie. Der Schmerz 2:125–143
8. Blumberg H, Jänig W (1983) Changes of reflexes in vasoconstrictor neurons supplying the cat hindlimb following chronic nerve lesions: a model for studying mechanisms of reflex sympathetic dystrophy? J Auton Nerv Syst 7:399–411
9. Carstens E, Klumpp D, Zimmermann M (1980) Differential inhibitory effects of medial and lateral midbrain stimulation on spinal neuronal discharges to noxious skin heating in the cat. J Neurophysiol 43:332–342
10. Casey KL (Ed) (1991) Pain and Central Nervous System Disease – The Central Pain Syndrome. Raven Press, New York
11. Cervero F, Morrison JFB (Eds) (1986) Visceral sensation. Progr Brain Res, Vol 67. Elsevier, Amsterdam
12. Chahl LA, Szolcsanyi J, Lembeck F (Eds) (1984) Antidromic vasodilation and neurogenic inflammation. Akademiai Kiado, Budapest
13. Chandler MJ, Brennan TJ, Garrison DW, Kim KS, Schwartz PJ, Foreman RD (1993) A mechanism of cardiac pain suppression by spinal cord stimulation: Implications for patients with angina pectoris. Eur Heart J 14:96–105
14. Chung JM, Fang ZR, Hori Y, Lee KH, Willis WD (1984) Prolonged inhibition of primate spinothalamic tract cells by peripheral nerve stimulation. Pain 19:259–275
15. Coderre TJ, Katz J, Vaccarino AL, Melzack R (1993) Contribution of neuroplasticity to pathological pain: review of clinical and experimental evidence. Pain 52:259–285
16. De Benedittis G, Di Giulio AM, Massei R, Villani R, Panerai AE (1983) Effects of 5-hydroxytryptophan on central and deafferentation chronic pain: a preliminary clinical trial. In: Bonica JJ, Lindblom U, Iggo A (Eds) Advances in Pain Research and Therapy, Vol 5, Raven Press, New York, pp 295–304

17. De Landsheere C, Mannheimer C, Habets A, Guillaume M, Bourgeois I, Augustinsson LE, Eliasson T, Lamotte D, Kulbertus H, Rigo P (1992) Effect of spinal cord stimulation on regional myocardial perfusion assessed by positron emission tomography. Am J Cardiol 69: 1143−1149

18. Devor M (1988) Central changes mediating neuropathic pain. In: Dubner R, Gebhart GF, Bond MR (Eds) Proceedings of the Vth World Congress on Pain. Pain Research and Clinical Management, Vol. 3, Elsevier, Amsterdam, pp 114−128

19. Dickhaus H, Pauser G, Zimmermann M (1978) Hemmung im Rückenmark, ein neurophysiologischer Wirkungsmechanismus bei der Hypalgesie durch Stimulationsakupunktur. Wien Klin Wschr 90:59−64

20. Dickhaus H, Pauser G, Zimmermann M (1985) Tonic descending inhibition affects intensity coding of nociceptive responses of spinal dorsal horn neurones in the cat. Pain 23:145−158

21. Dubner R, Ruda MA (1992) Activity-dependent neuronal plasticity following tissue injury and inflammation. Trends Neurosci 15:96−103

22. Duggan AW, North RA (1984) Electrophysiology of opioids. Pharmacol Rev 35:219−281

23. Edvinsson L, McCulloch J (Eds) (1987) Peptidergic mechanisms in the cerebral circulation. VCH, Weinheim

24. Fiallos-Estrada CE, Kummer W, Mayer B, Bravo R, Zimmermann M, Herdegen T (1993) Long-lasting increase of nitric oxide synthase immunoreactivity, NADPH-diaphorase reaction and c-JUN co-expression in rat dorsal root ganglion neurons following sciatic nerve transection. Neurosci Lett 150:169−173

25. Fields HL, Besson J-M (Eds) (1988) Pain modulation. Progr Brain Res 77. Elsevier, Amsterdam

26. Fu Q-G, Sandkühler J, Zimmermann M (1990) B-vitamins enhance afferent inhibitory controls of nociceptive neurons in the rat spinal cord. Klin Wochenschr 68:125−128

27. Galley D, Rettori R, Baccalon H, Medvedowsky A, Lefebvre JM, Sellier F, Chauvreau C, Serise JM, Pieronne A (1992) Spinal cord stimulation for the treatment of peripheral vascular disease of the lower limbs. A multicenter study in 244 patients. J Mal Vasc 17:208−213

28. Gebhart GF, Jones SL (1988) Effects of morphine given in the brain stem on the activity of dorsal horn nociceptive neurons. In: Fields HL, Besson J-M (Eds) (1988) Pain modulation. Progr Brain Res Vol. 77. Elsevier, Amsterdam, pp 229−243

29. Handwerker HO, Iggo A, Zimmermann M (1975) Segmental and supraspinal actions on dorsal horn neurons responding to noxious and non-noxious stimuli. Pain 1:147−165

30. Hanley MR (1988) Proto-oncogenes in the nervous system. Neuron 1:175−182

31. Hargreaves KM, Dubner R, Joris J (1988) Peripheral actions of opiates in the blockade of carrageenan-induced inflammation. In: Dubner R, Gebhart GF, Bond MR (Eds) Proceedings of the Vth World Congress on Pain. Pain Research and Clinical Management, Vol. 3, Elsevier, Amsterdam, pp 55−60

32. Herdegen T, Fiallos-Estrada CE, Bravo R, Zimmermann M (1993) Colocalisation and covariation of c-JUN transcription factor with galanin in primary afferent neurons and with CGRP in spinal motoneurons following transection of rat sciatic nerve. Mol Brain Res 17:147−154

33. Herdegen T, Rüdiger S, Mayer B, Bravo R, Zimmermann M (1994) Increase in nitric oxide synthase and colocalization with Jun, Fos and Krox proteins in spinal neurons following noxious peripheral stimulation. Mol Brain Res (in press)

34. Herdegen T, Tölle T, Bravo R, Zieglgänsberger W, Zimmermann M (1991) Sequential expression of JUN B, JUN D and FOS B in rat spinal neurons: cascade of transcriptional operations during nociception. Neurosci Lett 129:221−224

35. Höllt V, Haarmann I. Millan MJ, Herz A (1987) Prodynorphin gene expression is enhanced in the spinal cord of chronic arthritic rats. Neurosci Lett 73:90−94

36. Howe JF, Loeser JD, Calvin WH (1977) Mechanosensitivity of dorsal root ganglia and chronically injured axons: a physiological basis for the radicular pain of nerve root compression. Pain 3:25−41

37. Iadarola MJ, Ruda MA, Cohen LV, Flores CM, Naranjo JR (1988) Enhanced dynorphin gene expression in spinal cord dorsal horn neurons during peripheral inflammation: behavioral, neuropeptide, immunocytochemical and mRNA studies. In: Dubner R, Gebhart GF, Bond MR (Eds) Proceedings of the Vth World Congress on Pain. Elsevier, Amsterdam, New York, Oxford, pp 61−71

38. Jänig W (1988) Pathophysiology of nerve following mechanical injury. In: Dubner R, Gebhart GF, Bond MR (Eds) Proceedings of the Vth World Congress on Pain. Pain Research and Clinical Management, Vol. 3, Elsevier, Amsterdam, pp 89–108

39. Jänig W (1991) Sympathetic activity during peripheral nerve injury. In: Besson JM, Guilbaud G (Eds) Lesions of primary afferent fibers as a tool for the study of clinical pain. Elsevier, Amsterdam, pp 65–82

40. Kumazawa T, Mizumura K (1980) Chemical responses of polymodal receptors of the scrotal contents in dogs. J Physiol Lond 299:219–231

41. Larsson J, Ekblom A, Henriksson K, Lundeberg T, Theodorsson E (1989) Immunoreactive tachykinins, calcitonin gene-related peptide and neuropeptide Y in human synovial fluid from inflamed knee joints. Neurosci Lett 100:326–330

42. Le Bars D, Chitour D (1983) Do convergent neurones in the spinal dorsal horn discriminate nociceptive from non-nociceptive information? Pain 17:1–19

43. Le Bars D, Dickenson AH, Besson JM (1979) Diffuse noxious inhibitory controls (DNIC). Pain 6:283–327

44. Levine JD, Clark R, Devor M, Helms C, Moskowitz MA, Basbaum AI (1984) Intraneuronal substance P contributes to the severity of experimental arthritis. Science 226:547–549

45. Lewis T (1942) Pain. MacMillan, London

46. Lindblom U, Tapper DN, Wiesenfeld Z (1977) The effect of dorsal column stimulation on the nociceptive response of dorsal horn cells and its relevance for pain suppression. Pain 4:133–144

47. Lotz M, Carson DA, Vaughan JH (1987) Substance P activation of rheumatoid synoviocytes: neural pathway in pathogenesis of arthritis. Science 235:893–895

48. Lynn B (1977) Cutaneous hyperalgesia. Br Med Bull 33:103–108

49. Lynn B (1991) Silent nociceptors. Trends Neurosci 14:95

50. Maggi CA (1991) The pharmacology of the efferent function of sensory nerves. J Auton Pharmacol 11:173–208

51. Maier C, Waversik J (Hrsg) (1991) Schmerztherapie bei ischämischen Krankheiten. Gustav Fischer Verlag, Stuttgart

52. Meller ST, Gebhart GF (1993) Nitric oxide (NO) and nociceptive processing in the spinal cord. Pain 52:127–136

53. Mense S (1993) Nociception from skeletal muscle in relation to clinical muscle pain. Pain 54:241–289

54. Millan MJ, Czlonkowski A, Morris B, Stein C, Arendt R, Huber A, Herz A (1988) Inflammation of the hind limb as a model of unilateral, localized pain: influence on multiple opioid systems in the spinal cord of the rat. Pain 35:299–312

55. Mingoli A, Sciacca V, Tamorri M, Fiume D, Sapienza P (1993) Clinical results of epidural spinal cord electrical stimulation in patients affected with limb-threatening chronic arterial obstructive disease. Angiology 44:21–25

56. Morgan JI, Curran T (1989) Stimulus-transcription coupling in neurons: role of cellular immediate-early genes. Trends Neurosci 12:459–462

57. Myers RR, Yamamoto T, Yaksh TL, Powell HC (1993) The role of focal nerve ischemia and Wallerian degeneration in peripheral nerve injury producing hyperesthesia. Anesthesiology 78:308–316

58. Nahin RL, Hylden JL, Iadarola MJ, Dubner R (1989) Peripheral inflammation is associated with increased dynorphin immunoreactivity in both projection and local circuit neurons in the superficial dorsal horn of the rat lumbar spinal cord. Neurosci Lett 96:247–252

59. Nordin M, Nyström B, Wallin U, Hagbarth K-E (1984) Ectopic sensory discharges and paresthesiae in patients with disorders of peripheral nerves, dorsal roots and dorsal columns. Pain 20:231–245

60. Price DD (1986) The question of how the dorsal horn encodes sensory information. In: Yaksh TL (Ed) Spinal Afferent Processing. Plenum Press, New York, London, pp 445–466

61. Przewlocki R, Haarmann I, Nikolarakis K, Herz A, Höllt V (1988) Prodynorphin gene expression in spinal cord is enhanced after traumatic injury in the rat. Brain Res 464:37–41

62. Rang HP, Bevan S, Dray A (1991) Chemical activation of nociceptive peripheral neurones. Br Med Bull 47:534–548

63. Roberts WJ (1986) A hypothesis on the physiological basis for causalgia and related pains. Pain 24:297–311
64. Schaible H-G, Grubb BD (1993) Afferent and spinal mechanisms of joint pain. Pain 55:5–54
65. Sciacca V, Mingoli A, Maggiore C, Fiume D, Di Marzo L, Tamorri M, Cavallaro A (1991) Laser Doppler flowmetry and transcutaneous oxygen tension in patients with severe arterial insufficiency treated by epidural spinal cord electrical stimulation. Vasc Surg 25:165–170
66. Seltzer S, Marcus R, Stoch R (1981) Perspectives in the control of chronic pain by nutritional manipulation. Pain 11: 141–148
67. Seltzer Z, Tal M, Sharav Y (1989) Autotomy behavior in rats following peripheral deafferentation is suppressed by daily injections of amitriptyline, diazepam and saline. Pain 37:245–250
68. Stein C, Comisel K, Haimerl E, Yassouridis A, Lehrberger K, Herz A, Peter K (1991) Analgesic effect of intraarticular morphine after arthroscopic knee surgery. N Engl J Med 325: 1123–1126
69. Watson CPN, Tyler KL, Bickers DR, Millikan LE, Smith S, Coleman E (1993) A randomized vehicle-controlled trial of topical capsaicin in the treatment of postherpetic neuralgia. Clin Ther 15:510–526
70. Willer JC, Roby A, Le Bars D (1984) Psychophysiological and electrophysiological approaches to the pain-relieving effects of heterotopic nociceptive stimuli. Brain 107:1095–1112
71. Willis WD (1982) Control of nociceptive transmission in the spinal cord. In: Autrum H, Ottoson D, Perl ER, Schmidt RF (Eds) Progress in Sensory Physiology, Vol. 3. Springer-Verlag, Berlin, pp 1–159
72. Willis WD (1985) The Pain System. Karger, Basel
73. Woolf CJ (1984) Long term alterations in the excitability of the flexion reflex produced by peripheral tissue injury in the chronic decerebrate rat. Pain 18:325–343
74. Yaksh TL, Al-Rodhan NRF, Jensen TS (1988) Sites of action of opiates in production of analgesia. In: Fields HL, Besson J-M (Eds) Pain modulation. Progr Brain Res. Vol. 77. Elsevier, Amsterdam pp 371–394
75. Zieglgänsberger W (1986) Central control of nociception. In: Mountcastle VB, Bloom FE, Geiger SR (Eds) Handbook of Physiology. The Nervous System IV, Williams and Wilkins, Baltimore, pp 581–645
76. Zimmermann M (1977) Encoding in dorsal horn interneurons receiving noxious and non-noxious afferents. J Physiol (Paris) 73:221–232
77. Zimmermann M (1991) Central nervous mechanisms modulating pain-related information: Do they become deficient after lesions of the peripheral or central nervous system? In: Casey KL (Ed) Pain and Central Nervous System Disease – The Central Pain Syndrome. Raven Press, New York, pp 183–199

Author's address:

Prof. Dr. Dr. med. h.c. M. Zimmermann
Abteilung für Physiologie des Zentralnervensystems
II. Physiologisches Institut der Universität
Im Neuenheimer Feld 326
D-69120 Heidelberg
FRG

The endogenous neuromodulatory system

E. S. Krames

San Francisco Center for Comprehensive Pain Management, San Francisco,
California, USA

Since the first reports that electrical stimulation of the periaqueductal central gray
(PAG) in the midbrain of the rat [25, 32] produces profound antinociception, there
has been much progress in the understanding of the anatomical, physiological, and
pharmacological basis for an endogenous pain modulating system in animals and
man. It is the purpose of this chapter to review some of the seminal works and studies that have led us to our present understanding of this topic. The reader is advised
to read several of the excellent and more in depth reviews of this topic [5, 13, 15].

The demonstration that electrical stimulation of the midbrain central periaquaductal grey produces profound analgesia was particularly important to our understanding that there was, in fact, discrete anatomic endogenous systems mediating
and modulating, in a tonic way, the constant barrage of noxious information from
the environment. Specifically this demonstration first established that central modulation of the painful experience could be produced by anatomical areas other than
the cerebral cortex where pain is perceived and believed to be modulated by factors
other than nociception, including learning, behavior, and cultural influences.

This idea of a central modulation system for nociception, however, is not entirely
new. Prior to this demonstration, the observation that soldiers with massive war
wounds would often not feel pain during the initial shock of their injuries led careful
observers to believe that such a modulatory system existed. In 1965, citing these observations, as well as clinical studies on the seemingly paradoxical and painful results
of damage to afferent pain transmission systems, the "gate-control" theory of pain
was postulated [26]. Central to this hypothesis is that large myelinated fibers from
the periphery exert inhibitory control on the reception of pain from noxious stimuli
transmitted in small pain-carrying fibers through its inhibitory influences on a proposed dorsal horn "transmission" cell. Also inherent in this gate control hypothesis
was the suggestion of supraspinal modulation of pain through an efferent "central
control trigger mechanism".

**The anatomic and pharmacologic components of the neuromodulatory system:
The periaquaductal gray (PAG) to rostroventral medulla (RVM)
to dorsolateral funiculus (DLF) modulatory axis**

As stated above, the first neuroanatomic site found to be involved in pain modulation was the periaquaductal gray of the midbrain. As stated above, it was found that,
in rats, electrical stimulation of the PAG produced profound analgesia. This observation was later reproduced in man [23, 33]. Stimulation in all parts of the PAG produced analgesia, but several areas including the midline raphe dorsalis [29] and the

19

ventrolateral region of the PAG appeared to provide the most optimal sites for stimulation produced analgesia (SPA) [17].

Using the retrograde horseradish peroxidase technique, afferent projections to the PAG were localized to many areas of the forebrain, midbrain, and medulla including the medial prefrontal cortex, the basal forebrain, mesencephalic input from the nucleus cuneiformis and the substantia nigra, other midbrain structures including the nucleus subcuneiformis, the ventral tegmental area, the locus coeruleus, the parabrachial nuclei, and the hypothalamus. The medullary and pontine reticular formations, the medullar nucleus raphe magnus (NRM), and the superior central nucleus also supplied significant projection to the central gray. The hypothalamus was found to provide the largest descending input to the PAG [11].

The role for serotonin (5-HT)

Employing the tail flick test, the importance of cerebral monoamines in SPA of the PAG was studied in the rat [2]. In this study, depletion of all three cerebral monoamines, dopamine, norepinephrine, and serotonin (5-HT), by tetrabenazine led to a powerful inhibition of SPA which was restored by the injection of the monoamine precursors, 5-hydroxytryptophan (5-HTP) or L-DOPA. Depletion of 5-HT by *p*-chlorophenylalanine (PCPA) reduced SPA whereas elevation of 5-HT levels by injecting its precursos, 5-HTP, resulted in an increase in SPA. Likewise, dopamine receptor blockade with pimozide decreased SPA, whereas dopamine receptor stimulation with apomorphine and precursos elevation with L-DOPA, enhanced SPA. Unlike the above effects, selective depletion of norepinephrine with disulfiram actually caused an *increase* in SPA. These studies showed that dopamine and serotonin appear to *facilitate* SPA, while norepinephrine tends to *inhibit* it. it has also been shown that the most sensitive sites for SPA were found to lie in areas of the brain which contain 5-HT cell bodies such as the ventro-posterior PAG and the midline of the pontine and medullary brainstem including the nucleus raphe magnus (NRM) [30].

Evidence exists for a strong relationship between the supraspinal analgesia provided by opioids microinjected into the PAG and 5-HT. The PAG has been shown to contain both opiate receptors [4] and significant levels of endogenous opioid peptides [27]. Systemic naloxone reverses low threshold microstimulation of the rat medulla [38]. Microinjection of morphine into the PAG generates analgesia that is reversed by the injection of the opioid antagonist, naloxone, into the PAG [37], injection of the 5-HT antagonists, methysergide and cinanserin, into the PAG [36], and by lesioning the *dorsolateral funiculus* spinal projection pathway [28]. Microinjection of morphine into the PAG also alters activity in NRM cells responsive to 5-HT [10].

Evidence that an excitatory connection between the PAG and the NRM mediates SPA was generated by the observation that glutamate, when injected into the PAG of rats, caused both an increase in the firing rate of NRM and elevation of the flexion reflex threshold, which is a behavioral test for antinociception. Lesions of the NRM and its surrounding reticular area, specifically, the magnocellular reticular formation ipsilateral to the site of injection, abolished this rise in the reflex threshold. The authors concluded that increases in the activity of the cells in the PAG lead to analgesia which is mediated by the cells in the NRM and the adjacent reticular formation of

20

the rostroventral medulla [9]. Likewise, in a series of studies on anesthetized cats comparing the effects on spinal antinociception by SPA of the PAG and the lateral midbrain reticular formation by lidocaine blocking of either or both the nucleus raphe magnus and the lateral medullary reticular formation, it was found that it was necessary to block both areas before SPA could be prevented by the lidocaine [18]. Lidocaine blocking of either the medial or lateral medullary areas alone would not prevent the spinal antinicociception of SPA of the PAG. Thus, these observations support the notion that nociception is modulated through connections from the midbrain PAG to both the medial and lateral nuclei of the rostroventral medulla and then to the spinal cord.

Afferent connections of the rostral medulla in the cat were studied using the horseradish peroxidase (HRP) technique [1]. Iontophoretic injections of HRP were made into the midline and ventral NRM, the laterally located nucleus reticularis magnocellularis (Rmc), and the dorsally located nucleus reticularis gigantocellularis (Rgc). The predominant projection from the spinal cord to the medulla was found to be through the Rgc and no specific direct spinal projections to the NRM were found. Little distinguished the NRM from the Rmc. The major midbrain projection to the NRM and the Rmc derived from the PAG and the adjacent nucleus cuneiformis confirming this link between the PAG and the NRM. The Rgc received few afferents from the PAG. These authors concluded that "the demonstration of significant PAG projections to the NRM/Rmc provides anatomical evidence for the hypothesis that opiate and stimulation produced analgesia involves connections from PAG to 5-HT containing neurones of the NRM and Rmc which, in turn, inhibit spinal nociceptors." Furthermore, medullary connections from the RVM to the spinal cord through the dorsolateral funiculus have been extensively studied [6−8].

The role for norepinephrine

Although the excitatory influence of 5-HT on pain-suppressing mechanisms in the endogenous mudulatory system is well documented, the role of norepinephrine (NE) on modulation is less clear. As stated above, Akil and Liebeskind found that, while 5-HT and dopamine enhanced SPA in the PAG, NE inhibited SPA (antinociception) of the PAG. However, other studies have shown that NE has an inhibitory influence on nociception. It has been shown that both 5-HT and NE, applied iontophoretically to dorsal horn neurones, produce behavioral analgesia in animals [12, 21]. Also, administration of NE into the lumbar intrathecal space produced profound, dose dependent analgesia as defined by the tail-flick and hot-plate tests [31]. In this study, NE-produced analgesia was reproduced by phenylephrine and not isoproterenol and antagonized by the prior administration of the alpha-blocker phentolamine, but not propranolol, a beta-blocker. This is evidence of alpha-receptor, not beta-receptor mediation. Furthermore, in this study no cross-tolerance between intrathecal NE and morphine was observed, suggesting that the spinal action of morphine is not influenced by alpha-adrenergic terminals. These authors concluded that their data confirmed other reports that there existed a modulatory role of NE on the spinal transmission of painful information.

In a study utilizing direct recordings of wide dynamic range (WDR) postsynaptic neurones of either the spinocervical tract or dorsal columns of anesthetized and paralyzed rats, iontophoretically applied NE produced a potent selective inhibition of

21

nociceptive responses to heat or pinch, but no statistically significant change in the responses to innocuous brush or background activity [16]. This NE selectivity was mimicked by the $\alpha 2$-selective agonists clonidine and metaraminol, but not the $\alpha 1$ agonist phenylephrine, or the β-agonist isoprenaline. Furthermore, the $\alpha 2$ antagonists yohimbine and idaxosan either reversed or reduced the potency of the NE-elicited inhibition of nociceptive responses. These results, as in the Reddy and Yaksh study, strongly suggested that the $\alpha 2$ receptor mediates the selective inhibition by NE on WDR neurones of the spinal cord. Using immunocytochemical localization of retrogradely transported antibody to dopamine-β-hydroxylase following injection into the substance of the spinal cord and the retrograde transport of horseradish peroxidase, noradrenergic neurons which project axons to the spinal cord of the monkey were identified [35]. 79% of all NE containing cells with axons projecting to the spinal cord are located in the nucleus subcoeruleus and the nucleus locus coeruleus. No medullary cells were found to contribute to the noradrenergic innervation of the spinal cord.

The role for GABA

Most recently, there has been increasing evidence for GABA-mediated inhibition in the rostro-ventral medulla (RVM). In the rat, microinjection of the selective $GABA_A$ receptor antagonists, bicuculline and SR 95 531, produced a significant, dose-dependent increase in tail-flick latency which was antagonized by the $GABA_A$ receptor agonist THIP at the same site [22]. Administration of THIP resulted in a significant decrease in the tail-flick latency. These results suggested that a GABA-mediated process within the rostroventral medulla is essential for spinal nociceptive processing.

Rostroventral medullary neuronal specificity

Because specific neuronal populations fail to respond heterogeneously to excitatory experimental manipulations, confusion existed for the role of specific RVM neurones in the mechanism or mechanisms for neuromodulation. Specifically, most RVM cells are excited by noxious stimulation, but some cells are inhibited and some cells do not respond at all to stimulation. Actually, three classes of RVM neurons have been found [14]. These classes include the "on-cell," "the off-cell," and the "neutral-cell." The on-cell accelerates just prior to the tail flick response to noxious stimuli, the off-cell pauses just prior to the tail-flick, and the neutral cell shows no firing pattern when the tail flicks. The authors proposed that off-cells are the RMV-to-spine cells that inhibit nociceptive transmission since they pause just before escape mechanisms to nociceptive information take place. It is further concluded by the authors that SPA, opioid analgesia, or glutamate microinjection prevents escape mechanisms (analgesia) by preventing the off-cell pause. In other words, analgesic manipulation turns "on" the off-cell.

Spinal dorsal horn modulatory mechanisms

As previously stated, electrical stimulation of the PAG and the nucleus raphe magnus (NRM) produces analgesia by inhibiting responses to noxious stimuli of spinal dorsal horn neurons including those that give rise to the spinothalamic tract [19]. Likewise, the iontophoretic application of 5-HT inhibits activity of high threshold and wide dynamic range spinal neurons to noxious stimuli and glutamate pulsing [24]. The inhibition of primate spinothalamic tract cells by stimulation of the PAG or NRM is reversed or reduced after the IV administration of serotonin receptor antagonists. NRM stimulation is also known to inhibit the responses of dorsal horn cells to C fiber information [34]. The mechanism by which stimulation in the PAG or NRM inhibits dorsal horn neurons is thought to be due to presynaptic inhibition, however, stimulation of the NRM has als been shown to be due to postsynaptic inhibition [20].

In the PAG and rostroventral medulla (RVM), opioids activate and excite descending projection neurons, releasing inhibitory neuromodulators, while at the spinal cord level, they appear to inhibit the nociceptor directly through postsynaptic inhibition. Opiate receptor sites are also found on presynaptic afferents [4], however enkephalin terminals are not found on nociceptive afferent bodies or dendrites. Since, as stated above, intrathecal naloxone, microinjections of lidocaine to the RVM, and lesions of the dorsolateral funiculus reverses the analgesia produced by iontophoretically applied morphine to the PAG or stimulation produced analgesia of the PAG or NRM, it is clear that there exists an opiate link, presumably enkephelinergic, between the midbrain and spinal nociceptors.

Summary

In summary, the endogenous modulatory system for nociception derives from discrete anatomic structures from the forebrain, limbic system, and hypothalamic system to the dorsal horn of the spinal cord via the midbrain periaquaductal gray, rostroventral medulla, and dorsolateral funicular axis. Important neuromodulators for inhibition include serotonin from RVM cells, norepinephrine from the locus coeruleus and the locus sub-coeruleus, opioid peptides such as β-endorphin from the hypothalamus, enkephalins and dynorphin derived from large precursor molecules, and GABA, which appears necessary for nociceptive transmission. RVM to spinal dorsal horn cellular specificity through "on"- and "off"-cells in the RVM govern the tonic modulation of constant nociceptive barrage. Specifically, it appears that the "off"-cell is the cell which tonically inhibits this nociceptive information. Finally, opiate peptides at postsynaptic and maybe presynaptic terminals appear to inhibit nociceptors directly. This opiate inhibition may require serotonin, NE, or GABA to operate.

References

1. Abols IA, Basbaum AI (1981) Afferent connections of the rostral medulla of the cat: A neural substrate for midbrain-medullary interaction in the modulation of pain. J Comp Neurol 201:285−297
2. Akil H, Liebeskind JC (1975) Monoaminergic mechanisms of stimulation-produced analgesia. Brain Res 84:279−296
3. Atweh SF, Kuhar MJ (1977) Autoradiographic localization of opiate receptors in rat brain. I. Spinal cord and lower medulla. Brain Res 124:53−67
4. Atweh SF, Kuhar MJ (1977) Autoradiographic localization of opiate-receptors in rat brain. II. The brainstem. Brain Res 129:1−12

5. Basbaum AI, Fields HL (1984) Endogenous pain control systems: brainstem spinal pathways and endorphin circuitry. Ann Rev Neurosci 7:308–309
6. Basbaum AI, Fields HL (1979) The origin of descending pathways in the dorsolateral funiculus of the spinal cord of the cat and rat. Further studies on the anatomy of pain modulation. J Comp Neurol 187:513–532
7. Basbaum AI, Clanton DH, Fields HL (1976) Opiate and stimulus-produced analgesia. Functional anatomy of a medullospinal pathway. Proc Natl Acad Sci USA 73:4685–4688
8. Basbaum AI, Clanton DH, Fields HL (1978) Three bulbospinal pathways from the rostral medulla of the cat. An autoradiographic study of pain modulating systems. J Comp Neurol 178:209–224
9. Behbehani MM, Fields HL (1979) Evidence that an excitatory connection between the periaqueductal gray and nucleus raphe magnus mediates stimulation produced analgesia. Brain Res 170:85–93
10. Behbehani MM, Pomeroy SL (1978) Effect of morphine injected in the periaqueductal gray on the activity of single units in nucleus raphe magnus of the rat. Brain Res 149:266–269
11. Beitz AJ (1982) The organization of afferent projections to the midbrain periaqueductal grey of the rat. Neurosci 7:133–159
12. Belcher G, Ryall RW, Schaffner R (1978) The differential effects of 5-hydroxytryptamine, noradrenaline, and raphe stimulation on nociceptive and non-nociceptive dorsal horn interactions in the cat. Brain Res 151:307–321
13. Fields HL, Heinricher MM (1985) Anatomy and physiology of a nociceptive modulatory systems. Phil Trans R Soc Lond B 308:361–374
14. Fields HL, Bry J, Hentall ID, Zorman G (1983) The activity of neurons in the rostral medulla of the rat during withdrawal from noxious heat. J Neurosci 3:2545–2552
15. Fields HL (1987) Central nervous system mechanisms for control of pain transmission. In Pain, McGraw Hill, San Francisco, 99–131
16. Fleetwood-Walker SM, Mitchell R, Hope PJ, Molony V, Iggo A (1985) An $\alpha 2$ receptor mediates the selective inhibition by noradrenaline of nociceptive responses of identified dorsal horn neurones. Brain Res 334:243–254
17. Gebhart GF, Toleikis JR (1978) An evaluation of stimulation-produced analgesia in the cat. Exp Neurol 62:570–579
18. Gebhart GF, Sandkuhler J, Thalhammer JG, Zimmerman M (1983) Inhibition of spinal nociceptive information by stimulation in midbrain of the cat is blocked by lidocaine microinjected in nucleus raphe magnus and medullary reticular formation. J Neurophys 50:1446–1459
19. Gerhart KD, Wilcox TK, Chung JM, Willis WD (1981) Inhibition of nociceptive and non-nociceptive responses of primate spinothalamic cells by stimulation in the medial brain stem. J Neurophysiol 45:121–136
20. Giesler GJ, Gerhart KD, Yezierski RP, Wilcox TK, Willis WD (1981) Postsynaptic inhibition of primate spinothalamic neurons by stimulation in nucleus raphe magnus. Brain Res 204:184–188
21. Headley PM, Duggan AW, Griersmith BT (1978) Selective reduction by noradrenaline and 5-hydroxytryptamine of nociceptive responses of cat dorsal horn neurones. Brain Res 145:185–189
22. Heinricher MM; Kaplan HJ (1991) GABA mediated inhibition in rostral ventromedial medulla: role in nociceptive modulation in the lightly anesthetized rat. Pain 47:105–113
23. Hosobuchi Y, Adams JE, Linchitz R (1977) Pain relief by electrical stimulation of the central gray matter in humans and its reversal by naloxone. Science, Wash 197:183–186
24. Jordan LM, Kenshalo DR, Martin RF, Willis WD (1978) Depression of primate spinothalamic tract neurons by iontophoretic application of 5-hydroxytryptamine. Pain 5:135–142
25. Mayer DJ, Wolfe TL, Akil H, Carder B, Liebeskind JC (1971) Analgesia from electrical stimulation in the brain stem of the rat. Science 174:1351–1354
26. Melzack R, Wall PD (1965) Pain mechanisms: a new theory. Science, Wash 150:971–979
27. Moss MS, Glazer EJ, Basbaum AI (1983) The peptidergic organization of the cat periaqueductal grey: I. The distribution of enkephalin-containing neurons and terminals. J Neurosci 3:603–616

28. Murfin R, Bennett J, Mayer DJ (1976) The effect of dorsolateral spinal cord (DLF) lesions on analgesia from morphine microinjected into the periaqueductal gray matter (PAG) of the rat. Neurosci Abstr 2:946
29. Oliveras JL, Besson JM, Guilbaud G, Liebeskind JC (1974) Behavioral and electrophysiological evidence of pain inhibition from midbrain stimulation in the cat. Exp Brain Res 20:32–44
30. Oliveras JL, Guilbaud G, Besson JM (1979) A map of serotonogergic structures involved in stimulation producing analgesia in unrestrained freely moving cats. Brain Res 164:317–322
31. Reddy SVR, Yaksh TL (1980) Spinal noradrenergic terminal system mediates antinociception. Brain Res 189:391–401
32. Reynolds DV (1969) Surgery in the rat during electrical analgesia induced by focal brain stimulation. Science 164:444–445
33. Richardson DE, Akil H (1977) Pain reduction by electrical brain stimulation in man. J Neurosurg 47:178–183
34. Rivot JP, Chaouch A, Besson JM (1980) Nucleus raphe magnus modulation of response of rat dorsal horn neurons to unmyelinated fiber inputs: Partial involvement of serotonergic pathways. J Neurophysiol 44:1039–1057
35. Westlund KN, Bowker RM, Ziegler MG, Coulter JD (1984) Origins and terminations of descending noradrenergic projections to the spinal cord of monkey. Brain Res 292:1–16
36. Yaksh TL, Du Chateau JC, Rudy RA (1976) Antagonism by methysergide and cinanserin of the antinociceptive action of morphine administered in the periaqueductal gray. Brain Res 192:133–146
37. Yeung JC, Rudy T (1980) Sites in antinociceptive action of systemically injected morphine: involvement of supraspinal loci as revealed by intracerebroventricular injection of naloxone. J Pharmac exp Ther 215:626–632
38. Zorman G, Hental ID, Adams JE, Fields HL (1981) Naloxone-reversible analgesia produced by microstimulation in the rat medulla. Brain Res 219:137–148

Author's address:

Prof. Dr. E.S. Krames
Medical Director
San Francisco Center for
Comprehensive Pain Management
2299 Post Street Suit 205
San Francisco, CA 94115
USA

Some aspects on pathophysiology of pain in clinical angiology

H. Rieger

Aggertalklinik Engelskirchen, FRG

In general, there are many different receptors in the peripheral nervous system which, in principal, are divided into four main groups:

- Mechanoreceptors;
- Thermoreceptors;
- Chemoreceptors;
- Photoreceptors.

These receptors are highly specific and only respond when an appropriate, specific stimulus is applied. But there is one other type of receptor: the so-called nociceptors which show a reaction to a lot of different mechanical, thermal and chemical stimuli which finally lead to that what we call pain.

Pain can be elicited from many different tissues in the body. "Angiologic pain" comes from the connective tissue within the skeletal muscle and the muscle spindles, the skin, and the vessel wall itself.

The conducting nerve fibers and pathways belong to the Aδ and, mainly, to the C-group (Table 1).

Now, the problem of pains in vascular diseases should be discussed along with the clinical stage of disease. Thus, the first question is what about the pains in Fontaine stage II, or in other words: Which are the mechanisms of intermittent claudication?

Lewis studied in animal experiments the cause of pain which develops in a limb when circulation is occluded. From these experiments it is suggested that muscular activity releases a pain-producing factor (P) which passes out into the tissue spaces and is normally removed by the bloodstream. The substance accumulates, and when it reaches a certain concentration, pain develops. When the circulation is restored, the pain disappears within a few seconds.

Table 1. Classification of nerve fibers (Erlanger/Gasser)

Type	Function	$\varnothing$ (µm)	∇ (m/s)
Aα	– afferent and efferent motoric pathways to the skeletal muscle	15	100
Aβ	– afferent pathway of the skin for touching and pressure	8	50
Aγ	– motoric pathways to the muscle spindles	5	20
Aδ	– afferent fibers for T and *pain* of the skin	3	15
B	– sympathetic preganglionic	3	7
C	– afferent fibers of the skin for *pain*	0.5	1.0
	– sympathetic postganglionic (unmyelinated)		

These experiments explain the recurrent pain produced in the leg which suffers from peripheral occlusive arterial disease (POAD). Lewis's P-factor is still unidentified, but may consist of more than one substance, e.g.,

- lactic acid;
- potassium [k$^+$];
- adenine nucleotides;
- plasma kinines;
- protaglandines;
- different peptides.

Lactic acid and lactate

The general opinion is that lactic acid formation in muscle cells and its release into the surrounding tissue is the main factor for the stimulation of nociceptors and the development of pain. Of course, it is clear that lactate in working muscles increases. Experiments by Maas have shown that, in the healthy limb, lactate concentration normally increases by 497% under work load, and in the contralateral occluded limb by nearly 800%. The ratio between lactate and pyruvate was 14.3 and 26.3 at the end of exercise for the healthy and the occluded limb, respectively. If, however, lactate concentrations are really directly responsible for the development of pain in claudicants is, in may opinion, not completely clear.

We know some patients suffer from a so-called McArdle-syndrome. In these cases the formation of lactic acid is highly reduced or absent even under work load. In spite of that, claudication is possible!

The syndrome of painful muscle cramps with a failure of blood lactate to rise after ischemic exercise was first described by McArdle (1951). In these patients, we find an absence of phosphorylase in skeletal muscles. These types of diseases belong to the group of glycogenosis.

Potassium

More recent studies refer to the tissue concentration of potassium ions. We are familiar with pain arising along the vein during intravenous infusion of potassium-containing solutions. In case of claudication, the accumulation of lactate leads to a lowering of the pH value down to 7.1. For buffering, hydrogen ions of plasma pass into the cells and − to maintain the electro-chemical balance − potassium ions come out and pass into the tissue spaces where the nociceptors are waiting. Pain usually arises at a concentration of 15 − 20 mM/L.

The P-substances have not only the effect of direct chemical stimulation of nociceptors, they also more or less influence other receptors, e.g., mechanical ones, which become more sensitive to stimuli. This is the explanation for the clinical experience that pressing and palpation of muscles of claudicants is painful − even at rest!

Regarding the quality of pain in claudication, in general, most people describe pain in words which literally express how they feel their pain might have been produced. Most patients feel claudication as a cramping and tearing pain rather than as "pricking," "burning" or "cutting".

28

Now, we turn our attention to some *hemodynamic aspects.*

Whichever agent produces pain in claudication, the development and dynamics of pain depends on the ratio between the formation rate of P-substances, and the wash-out rate given by the remaining blood flow rate. If the remaining blood flow is high, which means a good hemodynamic compensation (collateralization), and the pain-free walking distance is long, the P-factors are quickly washed away and the rest period is short.

A special hemodynamic situation is the so-called *walking through phenomenon* in stage-II patients with a very good hemodynamic compensation of arterial occlusions. The *clinical* picture is the development of pain during walking which, however, does not force the patient to stop, but rather the pain disappears spontaneously when the patient continues to walk. The pathogenetic mechanism is as follows (Fig. 1): Within the initial period of walking there is a critical accumulation of P-substances which exceeds the threshold of pain. If walking is continued the vasodilatation of both the collateral and the muscle vessels enhance the wash-out effect. P-substances fall below the critical threshold of pain and the patient's walking distance is unlimited. This shows that the wash-out effect is an important pathogenic mechanism in claudication. If the wash-out effect is really an important point, its enhancement should lead to a lowering of ischemic pains and to an increase of the pain-free walking distance. Indeed, by *normovolemic hemodilution* blood flow can be enhanced both in macro- and microcirculation. Subsequently, the wash-out effect is enhanced and the pain-free walking distance tends to increase. As far as we know, the concentration of lactate acid and the lactic-pyruvate ratio, respectively, are only little influenced by moderate hemodilution. This indicates the major role of wash-out effect in development and control of claudication pains.

A new aspect concerning the development of claudication pains is the "Functional Compartment Syndrome." We recall the anterior tibial syndrome which is defined as

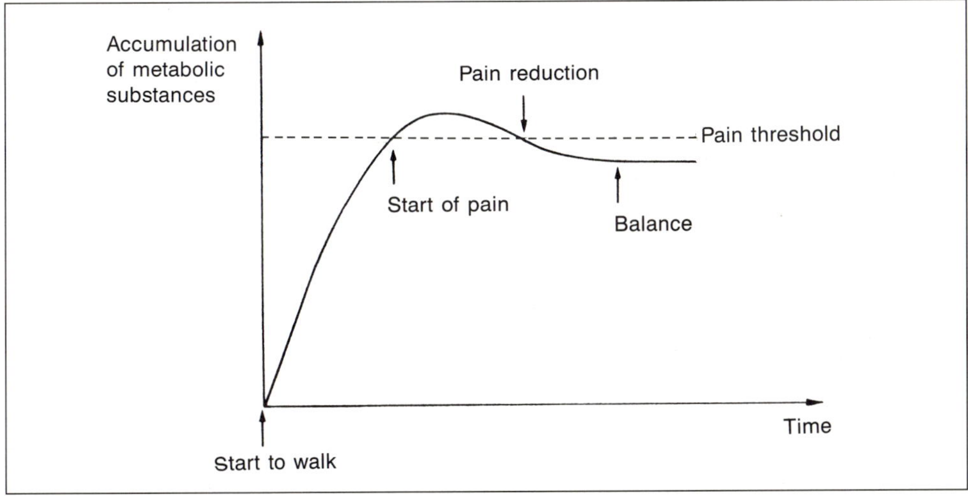

Fig. 1. After starting to walk it comes to a critical accumulation of P-substances which exceeds the threshold of pain (see first arrow). If walking is continued the wash out effect comes into play. P-substances fall below the threshold of pain (see second arrow) (from 2)

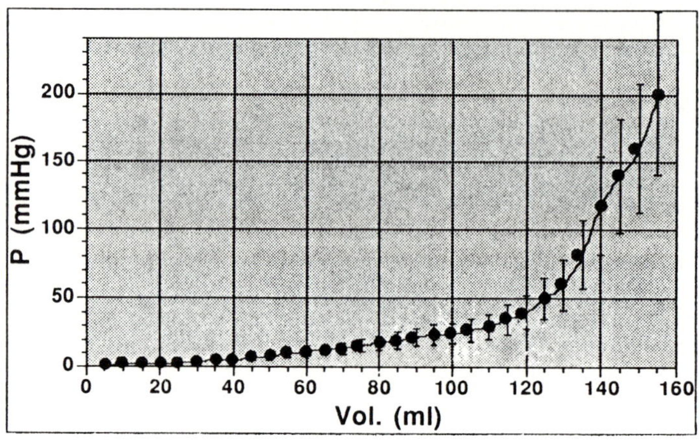

Fig. 2. Correlation between filtration rate and pressure within the fascial space (from 4)

a rise of tissue pressure for whatever reason within the fascial space of the tibial muscle. There are many causes leading to high pressure within the fascial space. One cause is a critical increase of muscle work during or after a strong march or jogging. In severe cases, muscle tissue becomes necrotic − the so-called 'march gangrene' which occurs even in healthy persons. The mechanism is that, during exercise, the transcapillary filtration rate is enhanced. As shown in Fig. 2 an increase of filtration volume up to around 60 to 80 ml does not change very much. From 80 ml on, however, there is an exponential increase of the tissue pressure within the fascial space.

There are three types of reaction during walking (Fig. 3): In *normal* persons the tissue pressure within the fascial tissue rises only to 40 mmHg at maximum. The second group, the so-called *intermediate* type, reaches a maximum of around 70 mmHg, and a so-called high *risk group* reaches 90 mmHg and does not decrease again with time. The *critical* threshold of tissue pressure is between 15 and 65 mmHg.

I believe that the mechanisms described here for the functional compartment syndrome could also be working in stage-II patients and probably are strongly involved in the development of muscle pains during walking. It could be that claudicants with a bad hemodynamical compensation belong to the risk group and that the muscle pains are not only due to the P-substances, but also to the increased tissue tension which follows the increase of filtration and tissue pressure. There are some arguments for this:

1) It is well known that in case of critical ischemia the permeability of capillaries is disturbed and enhanced respectively. The claudicant, however, is not endangered by a long standing critical ischemia, but the recurrent metabolic deficit could possibly also lead to an increase of the permeability of the capillaries involved, followed by an enhancment of subfascial pressure.
2) The pains suffered by the stage-II patients are exactly located as in those persons suffering from anterior tibial syndrome (Fig. 4).
3) The disappearance time of claudication pains in poorly compensated stage-II patients does constitute only seconds or a few minutes as is usual, but, rather 10 to 15 min or even longer − which is well comparable with the pains generated from anterior tibial syndrome in healthy persons.

30

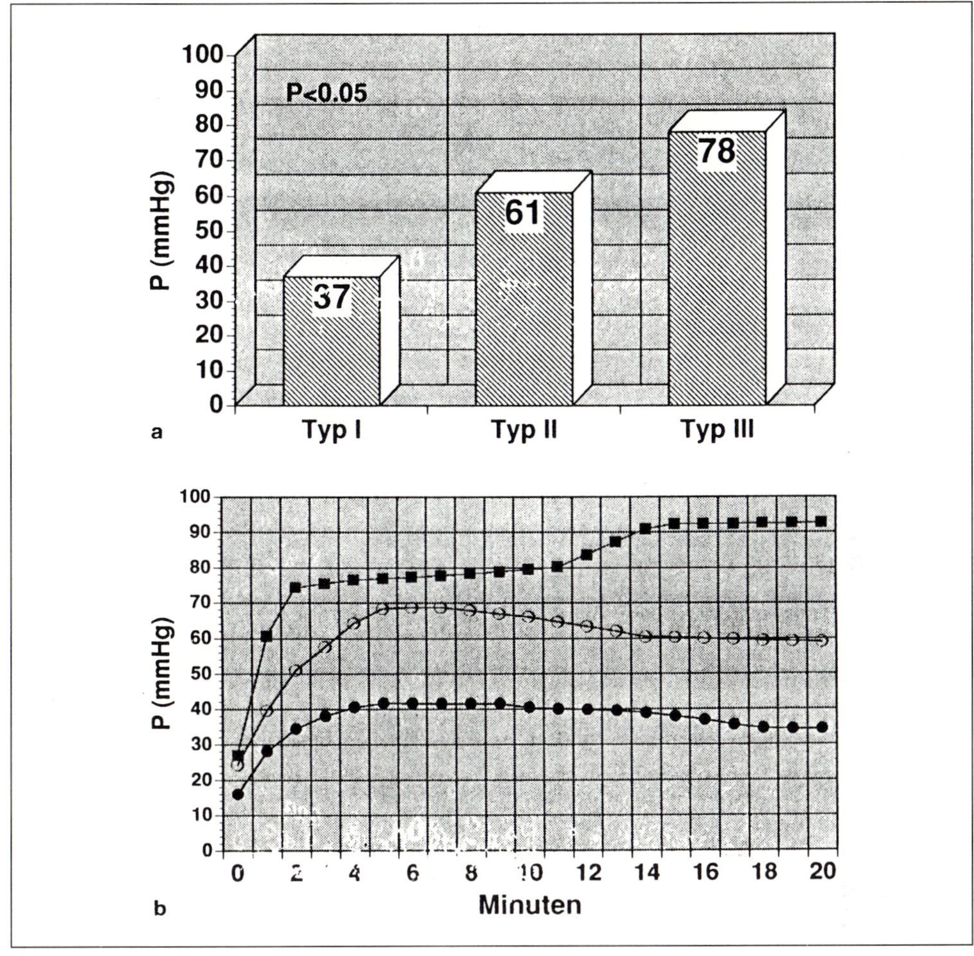

Fig. 3. Different types of pressure reactions during walking. ●————● type I, ○————○ type II, ■————■ type III (from 4)

Stage III

The Fontaine stage III of POAD is characterized by more or less chronic pain of the very peripheral areas of the limb, e.g., the forefoot. The explanation is that the perfusion has become so low that even the metabolites under rest conditions cannot be washed out in a sufficient way and induce pain. We should note that restpains usually develop in those areas of the limb which show the greatest distance from the heart. And just in these areas, like the forefoot, the skin represents the greatest part of tissue. We again note that skin perfusion at normal room temperature is only $3.0-10$ ml/min/100 g of tissue (under vasoconstricting condition even down to 1.0 ml/min/100 g of tissue). Thus, we can imagine that we need a strong reduction of skin perfusion for critical accumulation of metabolites which can develop rest pains.

31

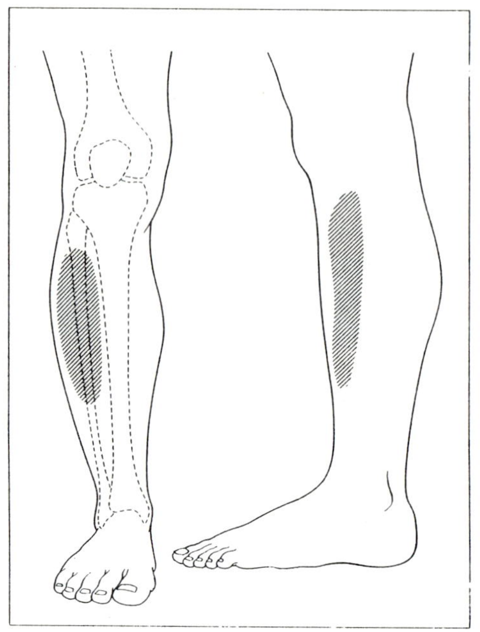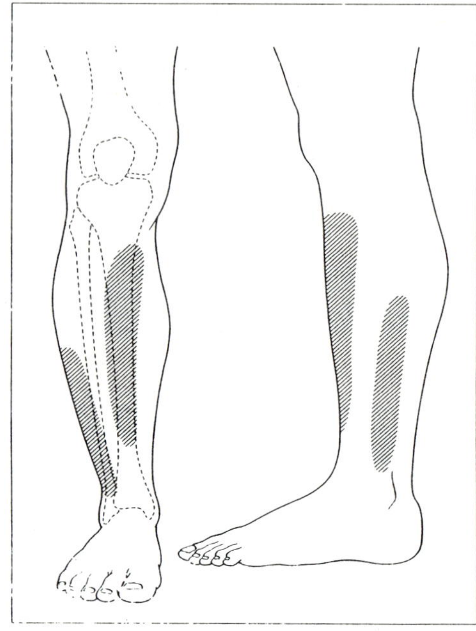

Fig. 4. Areas of pain diu claudications and patients with anterior tibial syndrome (from 4)

Typical for rest pain is the dependence on leg position. In horizontal position − above all, at night − the pressure difference between the heart/aorta and the foot is too low. Pain arises. After allowing the limb to hang down assuming a sitting position the hydrostatic pressure increases. This again induces the so-called Bayliss effect. This means that vessels which are out of the ischemic area show the normal response to pressure elevation: they vasoconstrict. Thus, a change in blood flow distribution towards those vessels occurs for those vessels already dilated for ischemic reasons. In other words: changing the limb position, e.g., hanging the limb down leads to a Robin Hood effect: "Stealing from the rich and giving to the poor". Therefore ischemic rest pain dissapears or improves.

Stage IV

In Fontaine stage IV of POAD another type of pain comes into play: the wound pain or the inflammatory pain.

It is often said that the pain of inflammation is due to increased tension in the affected issue. There may certainly be some increase of tension, but the most important factor is the reduction of pain threshold. That means hyperalgesia. The hyperalgesia may so enhance the effect of even normal stimuli that even arterial pulsation or something similar may be painful.

Inflammation is a cellular and humoral response to tissue injury by whatever noxes. In case of stage IV-patients the causing noxe is usually the ischemia itself that is responsible for necrosis of the corresponding tissue.

Both from the necrotic cells and circulating blood cells prostaglandins are released. The prostaglandins lead to a hyperalgetic state of pain receptors and to a lowering of the threshold of pains.

So, we come into a self-sustaining period of pain: Critical ischemia is painful because of the accumulation of pain-producing agents. Critical ischemia also leads to necrosis and release of prostaglandins and different peptides which in turn enhance the sensitivity for ischemic pain.

Thus, we can also understand a further clinical observation: If we apply PGE_1, sometimes ischemic ulcers become painful but not the surrounding tissue.

In spite of the strong relationship between the ischemic and inflammatory pain, we can separate them during everyday clinical work: Ischemic pains can be removed − at least for a certain time − if patients hang down the limb out of the bed. Pains by inflammation are enhanced!

What is the reason for that? During hang down of the foot the so-called Bayliss-effect comes into play, which I mentioned earlier. Pains become better or disappear. Inflamed areas, however, show an inverse effect: Pains increase probably because of a better blood filling of the cutaneous vessels. The warming-up effect of the tissue increases the formation of pain-producing metabolites.

Therefore another common observation can be explained: If the flow impediment of a stage-IV patient with local inflammation is removed, say by PTA, the diffuse ischemic rest pains disappear. The local inflammatory pains, however, increase!

If we look to treatment, we finally have three principal ways:

1) to enhance or to restore blood flow;
2) to treat the pains;
3) to treat the inflammation.

In many patients, we have to try all three. Whether or not and by which mode of action Spinal Cord Stimulation is one of these ways − needs further elucidation.

Author's address:

Prof. Dr. med. H. Rieger
Abteilung für Angiologie
Aggertalklinik
D-51766 Engelskirchen
FRG

Spinal cord stimulation in patients:
Basic anatomical and neurophysiological mechanisms

W. Jänig

Physiologisches Institut, Christian-Albrechts-Universität zu Kiel, FRG

A. Clinical observations and problems

Peripheral vascular diseases of the legs may lead to decrease of nutritional blood flow, ischemia, pain, ulcera, and other changes. These changes may eventually result in amputation of the extremity. Repetitive electrical spinal cord stimulation in these patients may lead to increase of blood flow through skin and deep tissues of the limb (in particular through the microvascular compartment) and of transcutaneous O_2-tension, may generate relief of ongoing pain (with increase of walking distance), and may be followed by healing of the ulcera (see Table 1 and contributions to this volume). This therapeutic intervention prevents amputation, at least in some of the patients, and improves quality of life. Interestingly, it does not appear to work in patients with autonomic neuropathy (e.g. in patients with diabetes mellitus) when the post-ganglionic axons are destroyed. Furthermore, the procedure is only successful, first, when the spinal stimulation electrodes are positioned over those spinal segments which contain the sympathetic outflow to the legs (i.e., in humans over the lower thoracic and two upper lumbar spinal segments) and, second, when the spinal cord stimulation generates paresthesias which are projected into the diseased limb.

In which way can the beneficial effects of electrical stimulation of the spinal cord be explained?

Table 1. Clinical situation

Spinal cord stimulation generates
- Increase of blood flow, in particular in the microvascular compartment
- Increase of transcutaneous O_2-tension
- Relief of pain (with increase of walking distance)
- Healing of ulcera

Can this beneficial effect be explained?
- Remote neural effect; possibly related to sympathetic innervation; unlikely to be primarily related to the afferent innervation
- Related to activity in postganglionic neurons which innervate the small resistance vessels
- Small diameter afferents involved because they can no longer dilate small blood vessels?
- Pain relief related to increase of blood flow (improvement of nutritional situation); are central mechanisms involved?

Supported by the Deutsche Forschungsgemeinschaft

1) It is very likely a remote neural effect and not a remote hormonal effect. It is
   related to the sympathetic innervation of the diseased extremity and very unlikely
   to the afferent innervation of the extremity. Antidromic activation of small
   diameter (myelinated and unmyelinated) afferent fibers generates vasodilation in
   skin and other tissues [5, 6]. However, it is very unlikely that afferent fibers are
   directly involved in the beneficial therapeutic effects of spinal cord stimulation,
   first, because the stimulation electrode is positioned 3 – 4 segments rostral to the
   segmental afferent inflow from the hindlimb and, second, because the patients do
   not experience severe pain during spinal cord stimulation. The latter would be expected to occur during stimulation of the afferent neurons with small diameter
   fibers.
2) The effect is associated with the activity (decrease, increase?) in post-ganglionic
   sympathetic neurons which innervate the small resistance vessels.
3) Small diameter afferent fibers may be indirectly involved. Normally, these fibers
   dilate small precapillary resistance vessels when they are excited (e.g., by noxious
   stimulation). In this way, they contribute, together with other mechanisms (see
   Fig. 1), to the regulation of the micromilieu. In patients with ischemia, these afferent fibers may not any longer be able to fulfill this function.
4) Pain relief following spinal cord stimulation is probably related to increase of
   blood flow (and therefore to the improvement of the nutritional situation of the
   micromilieu of the primary afferent terminal). It is unclear whether central neuronal mechanisms are additionally involved in the pain relief. After all, it is possible
   that the spinal cord stimulation inhibits transmission of nociceptive impulses in
   the dorsal horn and contributes in this way to pain relief.
5) All other changes which are observed in the patients during spinal cord stimulation are the consequences of the possible mechanisms mentioned.
   What is the state of our knowledge about the innervation of blood vessels and
   their neural regulation?

Remote and local control of blood vessels

Figure 1 summarizes the remote and local controls of blood vessels. The importance
of the different components is dependent on the type of blood vessels and the type
of tissue. Here, I want to concentrate on precapillary resistance vessels.

Remote control

1) All blood vessels are, with some exceptions, innervated by postganglionic
   noradrenergic vasoconstrictor neurons. Excitation of these neurons generates
   vasoconstriction.
2) Some blood vessels are additionally innervated by vasodilator neurons. Excitation
   of these neurons generates active vasodilation. Resistance blood vessels in skeletal
   muscle are innervated in some species by cholinergic vasodilator neurons; whether
   this is the case in humans is unclear [14]. Cutaneous resistance vessels probably
   are also innervated by sympathetic vasodilator neurons. The transmitter is unknown [14, 17, 41].

38

3) Pre- and postcapillary blood vessels in skin and subcutaneous tissues are innervated by afferent fibers. The fibers are unmyelinated (C-fibers) and thin myelinated (A-δ-fibers). Most of them have nociceptive function. Excitation of afferent C-fibers elicits precapillary vasodilation and postcapillary plasmaextravasation ["axon reflex"; 5, 6, 32, 43]. These functions could also be listed under local control of blood vessels. It is unknown whether different types of afferent C-fibers are differentiated with respect to these "efferent" functions. Excitation of A-δ-fibers may elicit precapillary vasodilation but no plasma extravasation [21].

4) Circulating substances (adrenaline from the adrenal medulla; hormones such as vasopressin released by the posterior pituitary gland, angiotensin II) may influence the blood vessels. Circulating catecholamines under physiological conditions, probably have little influence on small blood vessels, first, because the sensitivity of these blood vessels to catecholamines is too low; second, because the endothelial barrier to catecholamines in the blood stream is high [29, 30]. Under pathophysiological conditions this may change.

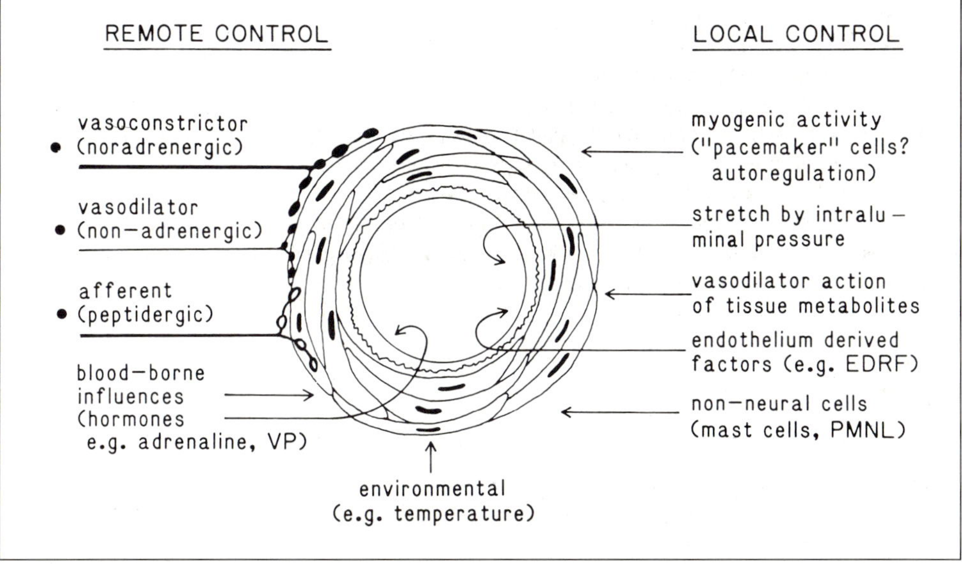

Fig. 1. Remote and local control of small arterial blood vessels. The remote control (left) is neural and hormonal. The neural control is mainly by noradrenergic vasoconstrictor neurons; some blood vessels are also innervated by postganglionic vasodilator neurons. Unmyelinated and A-delta afferent fibers may also be involved in the control by release of peptides (in this sense this neural control is more local). Blood-borne substances may act via the adventitial side or via the endothelium. For adrenaline the endothelium is a high diffusion barrier (see 29, 30). The local control consists of myogenic mechanisms and reactions to local mechanical stimuli, to tissue metabolites, to substances released by non-neural cells, and to endothelium derived factors. Furthermore, skin blood vessels may react to environmental influences (e.g., decrease or increase of temperature). EDRF, endothelium derived relaxing factor (which is identical to nitric oxide, NO); PMNL, polymorphonuclear leucocyte; VP, vasopressin

Local control

1) Smooth vascular musculature may develop myogenic activity and may react to stretch with contraction during increase of intraluminal pressure. This is the basis of the autoregulation of vascular beds. The mechanisms of the stretch sensitivity are poorly understood [28]. Stretch-sensitive ionic channels may be activated [1].
2) In some vascular bed, local tissue metabolites are important for the regulation of blood flow through arterioles. This process is particularly important in skeletal muscle. The changes in tissue metabolites (K^+, pH, adenosine, P_{CO_2}, P_{O_2}, phosphate, osmolality) during muscle activity may not only influence the vasculature but also the receptors of small diameter afferents [see 37, 38]. This may be particularly important under pathophysiological conditions.
3) The endothelium is important for the local regulation of small blood vessels [9]. An important substance is the "endothelium derived relaxing factor" (EDRF) which is identical to nitric oxide [NO; 42]. Shearing-stress applied to the endothelial cells by the intraluminal blood column leads to synthesis and release of NO which relaxes the vascular smooth muscle cells and dilates the blood vessels [1].
4) Substances released by non-neural cells in the micromilieu of blood vessels and afferent terminals influence the blood vessels. These substances are histamine (e.g., by mast cells), serotonin, prostaglandins, leukotrienes (e.g., by polymorphonuclear leucocytes, PMNL) and other substances. This may occur during tissue damage and inflammation.
5) Local changes of temperature may influence the small blood vessels and therefore the blood flow.

Changes of blood flow to stimulation of postganglionic vasoconstrictor fibers and of afferent fibers in normal and reinnervated skin

An animal model has been used which replicates many features of mixed nerve lesions with degeneration and regeneration of afferent and efferent nerve fibers. This may also occur in patients who develop microcirculatory disturbances and ischemic ("vascular") pain as a consequence of peripheral vascular disease (e.g., in diabetes mellitus). In the cat, the sural nerve (which supplies only hairy skin) and the tibial nerve (which supplies plantar hairy and hairless skin as well as deep somatic tissues) is cut and the proximal stump of the sural nerve is connected to the distal stump of the tibial nerve. After about 1 year or less, the fibers in the sural nerve have regenerated into the innervation zone of the tibial nerve. In this model, the reactions of blood vessels in the hairless skin of the central paw pad to an α_1-adrenoceptor agonist and to stimulation of the lumbar sympathetic trunk and of the peripheral cross-unioned nerve were studied using the laser-Doppler technique. In addition, functional reinnervation of sweat glands was studied using skin potential measurements and the iodine starch method. The experimental set-up is illustrated in Fig. 2. The following results were obtained [19, unpublished].

First, the blood vessels were reinnervated by postganglionic vasoconstrictor neurons. They exhibited normal or stronger than normal vasoconstrictions to electrical stimulation of the lumbar sympathetic trunk (Fig. 3 A lower trace control; Fig. 3 B lower trace experimental), although the density of innervation was at best about 30% of the control, as judged from the number of postganglionic neurons

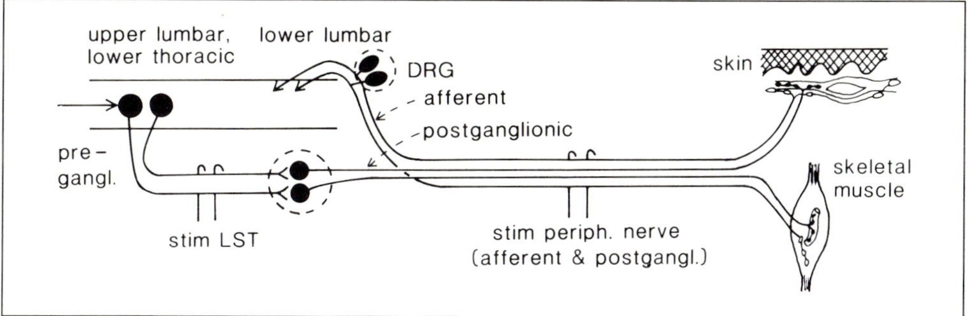

Fig. 2. Arrangement of stimulation electrodes for the experiments in Fig. 3

that project in the sural nerve relative to the number that project in the tibial nerve which includes the medial, lateral, and deep plantar nerves [36]. Furthermore, blood flow decreased after reflex activation of sympathetic vasoconstrictor neurons and increased after local anaesthesia of the sural nerve.

Second, systemic application of the α_1-adrenoceptor agonist phenylephrine produced a vasoconstriction which was much stronger in the reinnervated skin than in the control (Fig. 3 C). This is phenomenologically a clear sign of hyperreactivity of the reinnervated vascular bed.

Third, neurogenic vasodilation evoked by excitation of unmyelinated afferent fibers was almost absent in the reinnervated skin area, although a large proportion of the unmyelinated primary afferents had reinnervated the denervated skin area as judged from the activation of the afferent neurons by mechanical stimuli. Electrical stimulation of skin nerves always produced vasodilation in normally innervated skin (Fig. 3 A upper trace) indicating that the neurogenic vasodilation can override the vasoconstriction induced by simultaneous stimulation of postganglionic vasoconstrictor axons. Electrical stimulation of the cross-unioned nerve consistently elicited vasoconstriction in the reinnervated skin area (Fig. 3 B upper trace), indicating that the neurogenic vasodilation is considerably impaired. This may be due to a reduced release of vasodilator substances, to a defect in the release mechanism, or to a low afferent innervation density.

Fourth, sweat glands are readily reinnervated when the reinnervating nerve contains sudomotor axons.

These results show that the reinnervation of blood vessels by noradrenergic vasoconstrictor fibers and by afferent fibers is not normal. Is the innervation of the small blood vessels by nociceptive unmyelinated and myelinated afferents important for the regulation of the microvascular bed? Does the activity in these afferents interact with the noradrenergic postganglionic fibers? For example, it could well be that low frequency activity in polymodal nociceptive afferents which is ignored by the spinal cord and induces no sensations may affect blood vessels and interact with noradrenergic and non-neural components of the skin and other somatic compartments. Imperfect regeneration of afferent fibers following nerve lesions might then disturb the regulation of the microvascular bed. The same may also apply to the situation in patients with peripheral vascular diseases. It may be speculated that the vasodilator effect of small diameter afferents is reduced and the vasoconstrictor

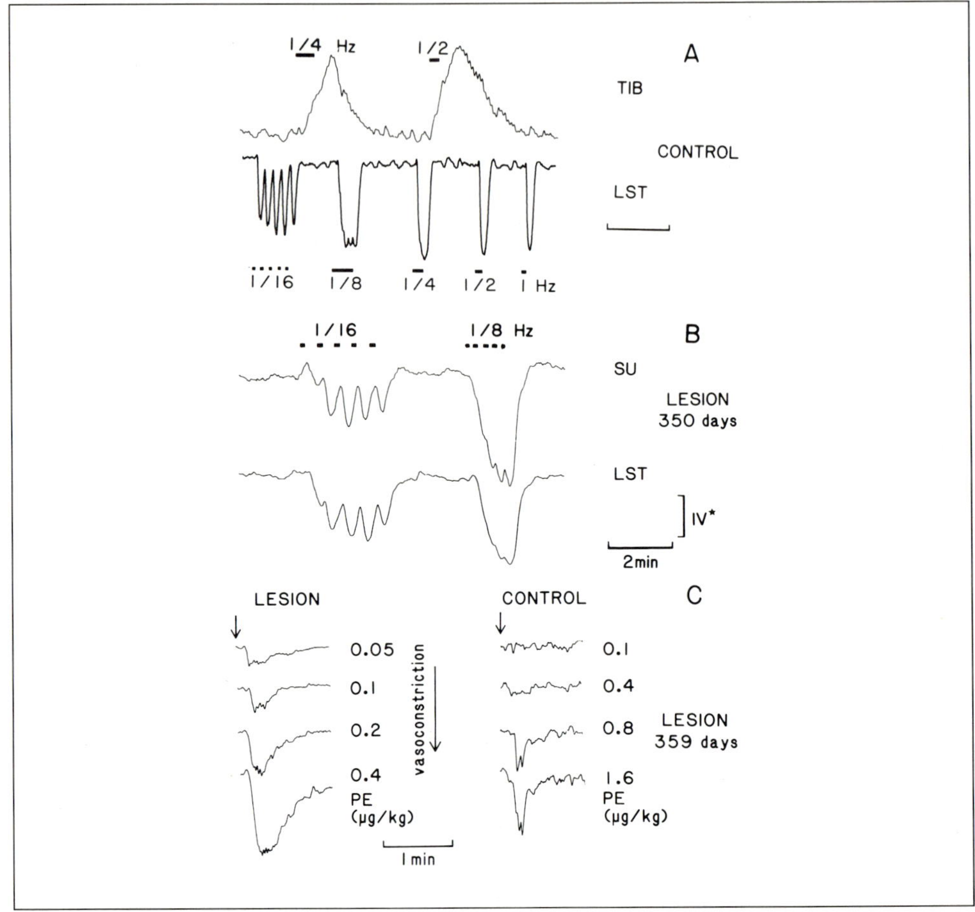

Fig. 3. Reaction of the blood flow through the dermis of the cat central paw pad (hairless skin) to nerve stimulation and to the alpha1-adrenoceptor agonist phenylephrine (PE) in control animals and in nerve-lesioned animals. The central stump of the sural nerve was cross-unioned to the perpheral stump of the tibial nerve about 1 year before the experiment. The plantar skin was reinnervated by the postganglionic neurons and the afferent neurons. Blood flow through the dermis was measured using a laser-Doppler flowmeter (time constant 1.5 s). The relative change of the measured flow is given as voltage readings (*V of the ordinate scale); the absence of flow corresponds to a value of zero. The nerves were stimulated at trains of 5 stimuli (0.062 to 1 Hz) and supramaximal strenghts: Lumbar sympathetic trunk (LST, preganglionic axons) at 10 V, 0.2 ms pulse duration. Cross-unioned sural nerve (SU, afferent and postganglionic) at 20 V, 0.5 ms. Tibial nerve (TIB, afferent and postganglionic; control) at 30 V, 0.5 ms. For position of stimulation electrodes see Fig. 2. A: Stimulation of TIB and LST in a control animal. B: Stimulation of cross-unioned SU and LST 350 days after nerve lesion. C: Injection of 0.05 to 0.4 (lesion, 359 days) and 0.1 to 1.6 µg/kg PE (control) into the jugular vein. (Jänig and Koltzenburg, unpublished observation; see also Jänig and Koltzenburg, 1991)

effect of vasoconstrictor fibers enhanced, leaving the microvascular bed "helplessly" exposed to this neurogenic vasoconstrictor influence.

Microscopic innervation of blood vessels and neurovascular transmission

Normal innervation

The mechanisms by which action potentials in sympathetic vasoconstrictor axons activate vascular smooth muscle cells and lead to reduction of blood flow through the blood vessels are at present still debated. It is commonly believed that noradrenaline released from the perivascular varicosities of vasoconstrictor axons bathes the adventitial surface of the vascular smooth muscle cells where it reacts with alpha-adrenoceptors to initiate vasoconstriction. This classical concept is based on two types of experimental observation:

1) Vascular constriction in response to exogenous noradrenaline and to trains of high-frequency stimulation of the nerve supply are largely abolished by alpha-adrenoceptor antagonist drugs.
2) Ultrastructural studies from random sections show that most varicosities of postganglionic axons lie at distances up to several µm from their target cells.

However, both these observations do not permit any conclusion about how neurovascular transmission functions during regulation of blood flow in vivo.

Morphological and neurophysiological experiments conducted recently have challenged the "classical" view and argue that the neurovascular transmission is morphologically as well as functionally specific, particularly to small diameter blood vessels (<200 µm in diameter). This concept is essentially based on two sets of experiments:

First, ultrastructural investigations of single varicosities of vasoconstrictor axons innervating small blood vessels using serial sections show that almost all varicosities devoid of Schwann cells form close contacts with vascular smooth muscle cells. The close contacts are morphologically like neuromuscular junctions. The basal laminae fuse, the vesicles in the varicosities which contain the transmitter(s) accumulate at the close contacts, and sometimes presynaptic specializations are seen [34, 35] (Fig. 4).

Second, neurophysiological experiments on small arteries in vitro show that stimulation of perivascular nerves with single pulses or short trains elicit excitatory junction potentials (EJP) and, in some arteries, small amplitude long-lasting potential changes (Fig. 5). The EJPs cannot be blocked by an alpha-adrenoceptor antagonist and may initiate action potentials (see upper inset in Fig. 5). They are either mediated by ATP released from the varicosities acting on subjunctionally located purinoceptors, or by noradrenaline acting on subjunctional "gamma"-adrenoceptors [4, 13]. The long-lasting potentials are mediated by noradrenaline and blocked by alpha-adrenoceptor antagonists, acting on receptors which are located extrajunctionally [12].

Although these in vitro results generated artificially by electrical stimuli which activate all axons synchronously are clear, it is not known how vasoconstriction is initiated by asynchronous activity of noradrenergic axons in vivo:

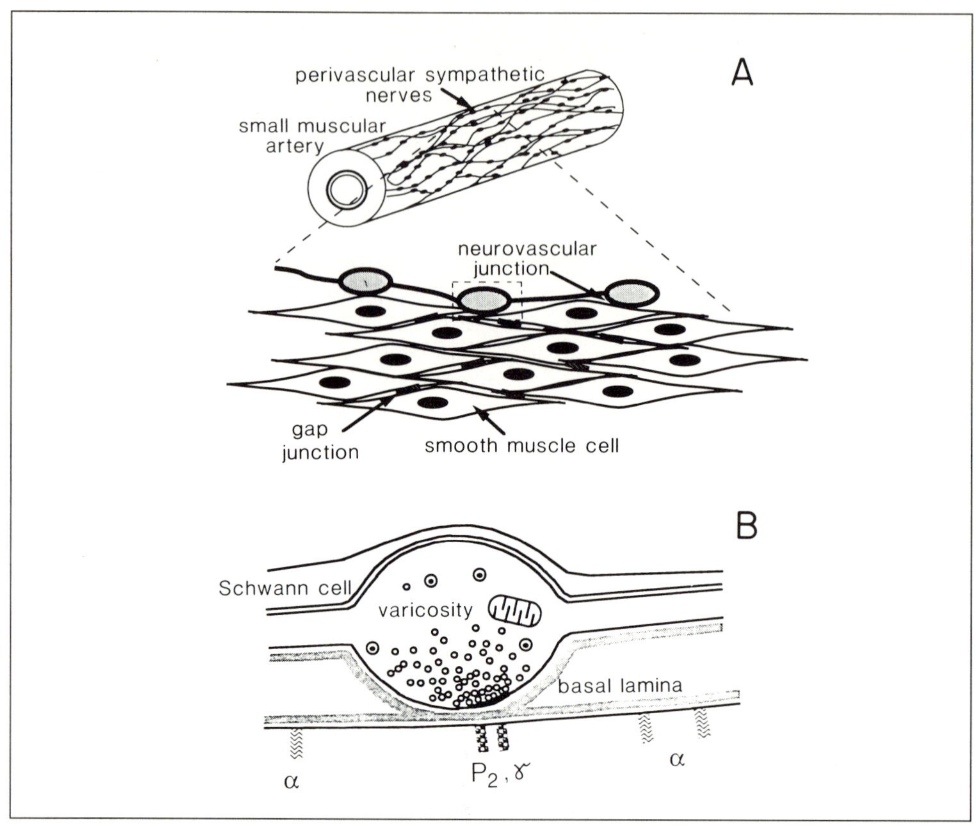

Fig. 4. The sympathetic neurovascular junction. A: Noradrenergic postganglionic vasoconstrictor axons form varicosities which contact the vascular smooth muscles from the adventitial side. Each vasoconstrictor axon has in the order of 10000 or less varicosities. Vascular smooth muscle cells are connected by gap junctions and form a functional syncytium. B: Diagram of the sympathetic neurovascular junction showing a varicosity with a presynphatic specialization and accumulation of synaptic vesicles. These synaptic vesicles contain noradrenaline and ATP. Some large granular vesicles also contain neuropeptide Y. Activation of the postganglionic vasoconstrictor neuron leads to release of quanta from vesicles at the junction. These quanta activate postsynaptic (subjunctional) receptors of the vascular smooth muscle cells, which are either purinergic receptors (P_2-purinoceptors for ATP) or gamma-adrenoceptors (for details see Hirst and Edwards, 1989). At sites removed from the junction itself, alpha-adrenoceptors may be affected by noradrenaline diffusing from the terminals, or by exogeneous catecholamines. A and B from Jobling, unpublished

1) It appears that the effects of EJPs may be particularly important for the small blood vessels (small arterioles and possibly venules in skin); these vessels regulate the micromilieu of the receptive terminals of the nociceptive neurons. In arterioles the neurogenic alpha-depolarization is not detected [13, 26] and constriction is not mediated via alpha-adrenoceptors [8].

2) Circulating catecholamines under physiological conditions probably have little influence on small blood vessels because a) their sensitivity to noradrenaline is too low; b) the endothelial barrier to catecholamines and other substances in the

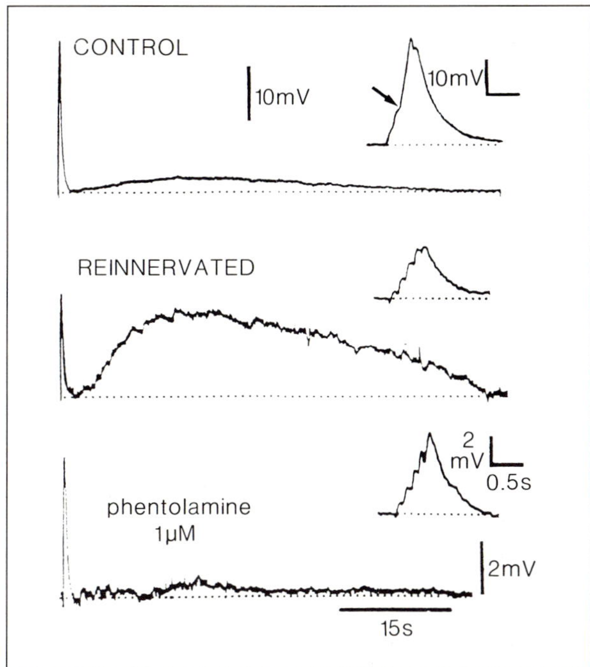

Fig. 5. Responses evoked in smooth muscle cells of the rat tail artery to supramaximal electrical stimuli applied to the perivascular nerves in controls and in reinnervated preparations. Excitatory junction potentials (EJP) and neurogenic alpha-adrenoceptor mediated depolarizations evoked in the smooth muscle cells in response to 5 supramaximal stimuli at 10 Hz applied to the perivascular nerves (see upper part of Fig. 4). The insets show the junction potentials on an expanded time scale. In the control preparation, an action potential is initiated during the train (see arrow in upper inset) and is followed by an alpha-depolarization of 2 mV amplitude. Early in reinnervation (24 day p.o.), the EJPs are very small (see also lower inset), but the alpha-depolarization is relatively large. In the lower trace phentolamine (alpha-adrenoceptor antagonist) is added to the superfusate. The alpha-depolarization is abolished without affecting the EJP. (Modified from Jobling et al. 1992)

blood stream is high [29, 30, see Fig. 1], and c) because the concentration gradient of catecholamines near the arterioles is probably away from the adventitial side toward the venules as most of the circulating noradenaline comes from nerve terminals [7]. Do EJPs and neurogenic alpha-depolarizations interact in the generation of vasoconstriction? Does noradrenaline, which is released from the varicosities during tonic activity in the vasoconstrictor neurons, reach a high enough concentration to interact with the extrajunctional alpha-adrenoceptors leading to vasoconstriction without membrane potential changes?

3) Varicosities of vasoconstrictor axons do not only release noradrenaline and ATP, but also neuropeptides (such as neuropeptide Y) which is present in the large granular vesicles (see Fig. 4B). These peptides are commonly referred to as transmitters. However, it is unclear what biological effects these neuropeptides have on the blood vessels, although neuropeptide Y is known to potentiate contraction independently of membrane potential changes [39, 40].

Although the way in which arterial vessels are normally controlled by nerves is not well understood, a number of these aspects of neuroeffector control have been examined in arterial vessels after reinnervation.

Neurovascular transmission after regeneration

As mentioned above, when sural axons reinnervated the plantar skin in the cat, vasoconstrictor responses to nerve stimulation were enhanced relative to normal, and hyperreactivity to exogenous catecholamines was present after the functional innervation had returned [19]. Electrophysiological and histochemical studies on the rat tail artery [27] have revealed a similar abnormal situation at sites of neurovascular interaction following regeneration of the original innervation. When the major nerve trunks which carry the postganglionic noradrenergic axons supplying the tail artery were briefly frozen, so as to disrupt the axons with minimal interference to their Schwann cells and the perineurium, there was initially rapid regeneration (1 – 2 mm/day), and functional perivascular axons could be demonstrated about 50 mm distal to the lesion site after about 50 days. Intracellular recordings demonstrated small EJPs followed by relatively large nerve-mediated alpha-depolarizations (Fig. 5, lower records). At this stage a patchy distribution of varicose noradrenergic axons had returned to the outer surface of the artery at this location, although no axons were in contact with the artery at distal sites (> 70 mm) where perivascular stimuli failed to evoke any electrical response in the vascular smooth muscle. After longer periods of 100 – 120 days, the mean EJP amplitude became comparable to that in age-matched controls. The alpha-depolarization also increased in amplitude and remained larger than in controls as long as the studies were made. However, at distances > 100 mm along the tail artery there was little or no evidence of any functional innervation even after the longest period (140 days).

The histochemical picture confirmed these observations. Although the recovery of EJPs paralleled the redevelopment of a perivascular plexus in the proximal half of the denervated artery, the artery was rarely reinnervated at all at distal sites even after 200 days post-lesion. Furthermore, image analysis of the regenerated plexus at proximal sites revealed that it contained less than 85% as much noradrenaline as paired control material (McLachlan, unpublished observation). The failure to reinnervate the artery more than 7 – 9 cm beyond the lesion was quite specific as the adjacent arterio-venous anastomoses in the distal half of the tail became completely reinnervated within < 100 days, and brightly fluorescent axon bundles could be seen within nerve trunks at the tip of the tail apparently growing past the denervated artery. In the distal tail skin of the same animals, there was also a paucity of fine axons containing the neuropeptides Substance P and CGRP (McLachlan and Keast, unpublished).

These data show that neurovascular transmission, at least of the cutaneous vessels which have been studied in these experiments, does not recover to its original state after the perivascular axons have degenerated. In fact the vascular smooth muscle remains modified after denervation so that the conductance change produced by what are probably reduced amounts of noradrenaline acting on alpha 2-adrenoceptors is potentiated even after the innervation is reestablished. It seems possible that there may be hyperreactivity to neurally-evoked vasoconstriction mediated via alpha 1-adrenoceptors (i.e., non-electrogenic constriction), leading to the enhanced

46

responses seen in the cross-innervated cat plantar skin [19]. Similar changes may occur in patients with peripheral vascular diseases and patients with diabetes mellitus who develop neuropathies of postganglionic and sensory fibers with degeneration and regeneration of these fibers to their target tissues.

Physiological impulse activity in postganglionic neurons innervating blood vessels

A general idea about the organization of the sympathetic nervous system

Activity is transmitted from the spinal cord to the target organs by discrete pathways which consist of pre- and postganglionic neurons and constitute the final common sympathetic pathways to the periphery (Fig. 6). In neurophysiological experiments on cats, groups of pre- and postganglionic neurons have been found to behave precisely as predicted from the reflex responses of the target tissues. These reflex responses are elicited by appropriate physiological stimuli exciting arterial baro- and chemoreceptors, other visceral receptors, various types of cutanous receptors, etc.

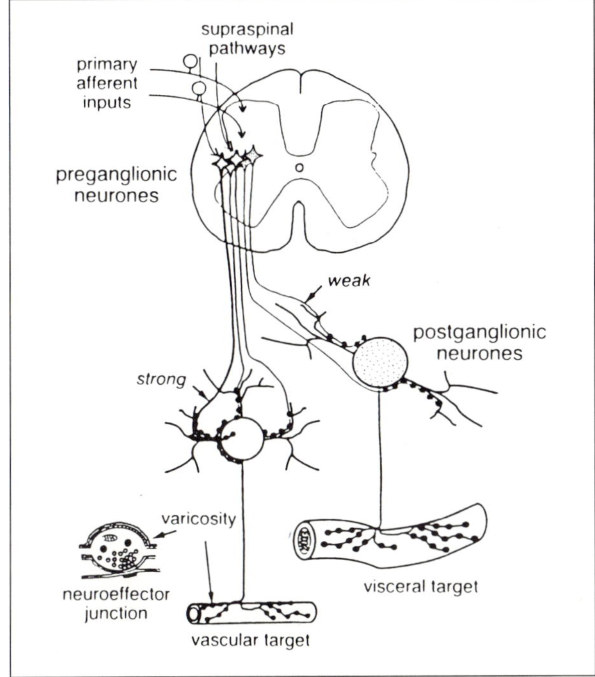

Fig. 6. Organization of the sympathetic nervous system in building blocks. Separate functional pathways exist from within the CNS to the effector organs. Preganglionic neurons located in the intermediate zone integrate signals descending from brain stem and hypothalamus and arising segmentally from primary afferent fibers. The preganglionic neurons project to peripheral ganglia and converge onto postganglionic neurons. Some preganglionic synaptic inputs to postganglionic neurons in paravertebral ganglia and to some postganglionic neurons in prevertebral ganglia are strong and are always suprathreshold. The postganglionic axons form multiple neuroeffector junctions with their target cells. (From Jänig and McLachlan, 1992)

The reflex responses characterize the pre- and postganglionic neurons as belonging to a particular pathway and are functional "fingerprints" (markers) of that pathway. Figure 7 demonstrates, as an example, reflexes in muscle vasoconstrictor (MVC) neurons, cutaneous vasoconstrictor (CVC) neurons and sudomotor (SM) neurons projecting to the cat hindlimb, under standardized experimental conditions. These reflex responses are the expression of the organization of the sympathetic system in the periphery and in the spinal cord, brain stem, and hypothalamus [14, 15].

So far, 12 different functional groups of sympathetic neurons have been identified in the lumbar sympathetic outflow to skin, skeletal muscle, pelvic viscera, and in the sympathetic outflow to the head and the upper neck. Many neurons of eight of these pathways have continuous (ongoing) activity such as most muscle vasoconstrictor neurons, cutaneous vasoconstrictor neurons, and sudomotor neurons (see Fig. 7).

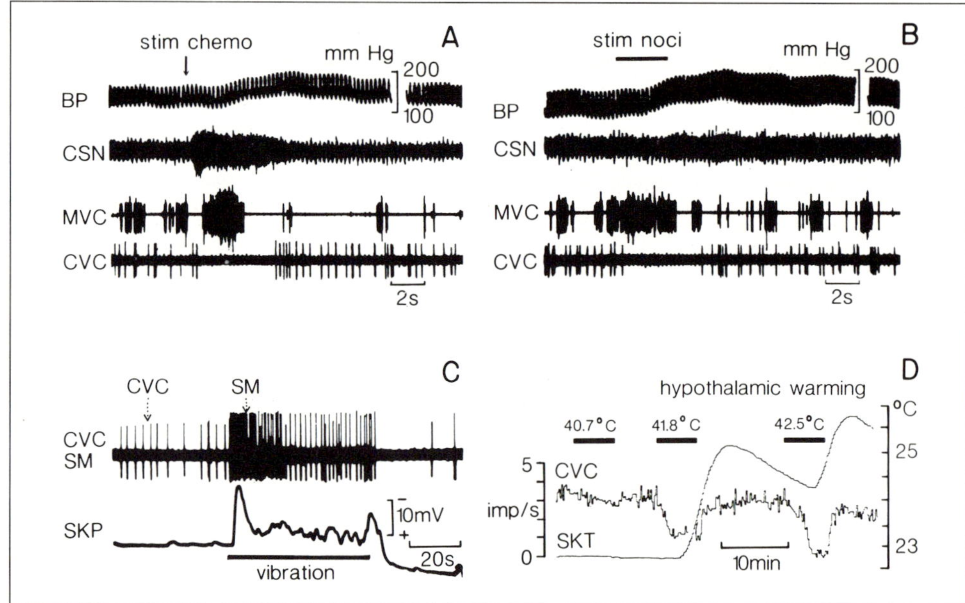

Fig. 7. Reflexes in muscle (MVC) and cutaneous (CVC) vasoconstrictor and sudomotor (SM) neurons recorded from postganglionic axons in anesthetized cats. A. Stimulation of the carotid chemoreceptors by a retrograde bolus injection of 0.2 ml CO_2-enriched saline into the lingual artery (indicated by arrow) activated the MVC neurons and depressed the CVC neuron which were simultaneously recorded. The stimulus was controlled by recording the afferent activity in the carotid sinus nerve (CSN). The increase of blood pressure evoked by chemoreceptor stimulation led to a baroreceptor mediated depression of the MVC neurons but not of the CVC neuron. B. Stimulation of cutaneous nociceptors by pinching the ipsilateral hindpaw (indicated by bar) also excited by MVC neurons and inhibited the CVC neuron. C. Simultaneous recording of a single CVC neuron (small signal) and a single SM neurone (larger signal) and the skin potential from the central paw pad. Stimulation of Pacinian corpuscles by vibration excited the SM neuron and inhibited the CVC neuron. SM activation was correlated with the negative deflections of the skin potential (SKP). D. Inhibition of CVC neurons to warming of the anterior hypothalamus. Note the increase of skin temperature (SKT), measured on the central paw pad, which followed the depression of CVC activity. (Data for A–C from Jänig and Kümmel, unpublished; for D from Jänig, 1985. From Jänig and McLachlan, 1992)

The ongoing activity in these types of neurons exhibits typical fluctuations with the central respiration, and this respiratory profile is characteristic for each type of neuron, indicating distinct central coupling between regulation of respiration and sympathetic systems [10]. Other types of neurons are silent and can only be activated by central stimuli, probably only during very specific behavioral constellations [for review see 14, 15, 16, 22, 23].

Sympathetic pathways to skin and skeletal muscle

Figure 8 shows the sympathetic pathways which innervate skeletal muscle and skin of the hindlimb. Three of the systems have ongoing activity (systems in black in Fig. 8). This depends, in the CVC and SM neurons, on the thermoregulatory state of the organism, but not in the MVC neurons. The other systems are normally probably silent. It is likely that the number of distinct sympathetic pathways innervating these somatic target tissues is higher. For example, different sections of the cutaneous vascular bed (precapillary resistance (nutritional) vessels, postcapillary capacitance vessels (veins), arterio-venous anastomoses) may each have a separate sympathetic innervation; furthermore, in humans, the skin of the cutaneous vasoconstrictor supply of the distal parts of the extremities (hands and feet) may be different from the cutaneous vasoconstrictor supply of the more proximal skin and of the trunk. Finally, "non-classical" target organs may have a separate sympathetic innervation, such as the skin-associated lymphoid tissue and the fat tissue.

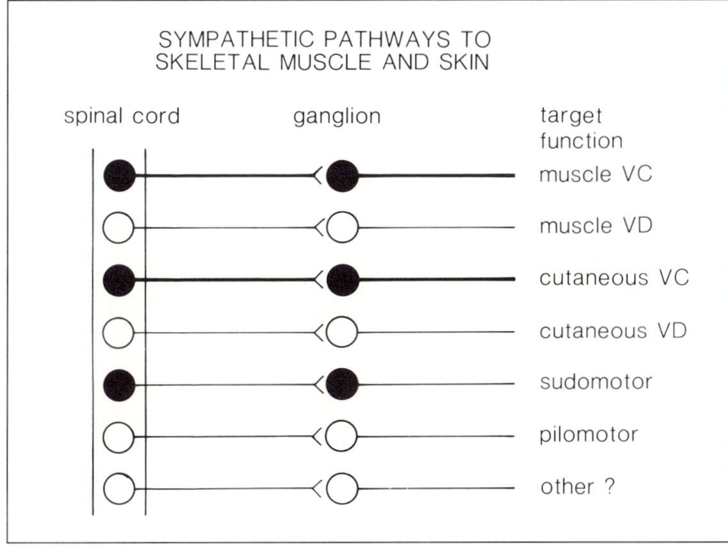

Fig. 8. Functional types of sympathetic pathways to skin and skeletal muscle. In black pathways with ongoing activity. Neurons of the other pathways are normally silent

Which mechanisms operate during spinal cord stimulation?

Idea that sympathetic outflow is involved is supported by animal experiments

Linderoth et al. (1989) have conducted experiments on anesthetized rats showing that repetitive electrical dorsal column stimulation increases the blood flow in the plantar skin of the hindpaw (Fig. 9 A). A pair of stimulation electrodes was positioned above the dorsal columns at the segmental level of Tl3 − L1. The stimulation parameters were similar to those used in patients with peripheral vascular disease. The blood flow through the skin was measured with a laser Doppler flowmeter. The cutaneous blood flow first increased and then decreased to a steady state level which was > 30% above the base line before the stimulation. The increase of blood flow outlasted the end of the stimulus train by several 10 s. In some animals the authors were not able to elicit an increase of blood flow through the skin by the spinal cord stimulation although the control parameters were identical. These negative results may well be related to the depth of anesthesia because the vasoconstrictor activity is depressed under pentobarbital anesthesia.

The hindlimb of the rat is innervated by lumbar afferent neurons of the segments L4 and L5. Repetitive electrical stimulation of the distal stumps of the sectioned dorsal roots L4 and L5 at strength which probably only excited myelinated fibers did not induce a vasodilation in the plantar skin (lower record in Fig. 9 B). When the stimulus strength was increased, so as to excite the unmyelinated afferent fibers, a cutaneous vasodilation was observed. Electrical stimulation of the proximal stump

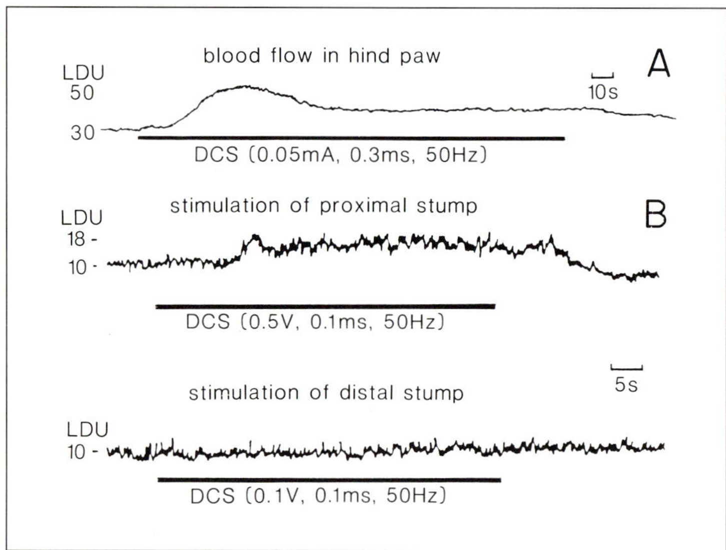

Fig. 9. Skin blood flow in a rat hindpaw during repetitive electrical stimulation of the ipsilateral dorsal column (A) or during repetitive electrical stimulation of the proximal or distal stump of the sectioned dorsal roots innervating the hind paw (B). Stimulus strength, duration and frequencies are indicated. The blood flow was measured with a laser Doppler flowmeter in LDU (laser Doppler arbitrary units). (Modified from Linderoth et al. (1989), with permission)

of the dorsal roots L 4 and L 5 generated a slight increase in blood flow (upper record in Fig. 9 B). These results argue that the sympathetic outflow is involved in the increase of blood flow. Later, the authors have shown that sympathectomy alleviated the increase of blood flow during spinal cord stimulation (Linderoth and coworkers, unpublished). These experiments are preliminary and must be repeated under more controlled experimental conditions which include recordings from sympathetic neurons (see below).

The spinal cord contains neural circuits which generate inhibition in vasoconstrictor activity

Noxious stimulation of skin (by radiant heat and mechanical) elicits well-defined reflexes in cutaneous vasoconstrictor (CVC) neurons in standardized experimental conditions. These reflexes were first described by Lovén (1866) in rabbits. For the CVC neurones supplying the cat and rat skin of the hindlimb or the head of the cat, this reflex is preferentially elicited by noxious stimulation of the ipsilateral skin, which is innervated by the CVC neurones; however, it is weak or absent when the skin on the contralateral body side is stimulated (Fig. 10 A). Reflexes in muscle vasoconstrictor (MVC) neurons (Fig. 10 B) and sudomotor neurons do not exhibit this spatial organization when noxious stimuli are applied to the skin of the paws of different extremities [3, 14, 15]. In unanaesthetized humans the inhibitory reflex in CVC neuron upon noxious stimulation of skin cannot be elicited since noxious stimuli generate arousal reactions and, consequently, an activation of the CVC neurons [cf. 25]. This is probably equivalent to the defense reaction. Recent investigations on humans have shown that electrical intraneural stimulation of thin myelinated afferents in skin nerves of the foot elicits reflex dilatation (increase of blood flow) in skin areas lying adjacent to or in the territory of the stimulated nerve (Blumberg and Wallin 1987). The dilatation in the skin was abolished by blockade of the conduction in the nerve proximal to the stimulation site. It was largest in the skin of the stimulated foot and smaller on the contralateral foot. Thus, the reflex in humans appears to be very similar to the inhibitory reflex in CVC neurons elicited by cutaneous noxious stimuli in anesthetized cats and rats (see Fig. 10 A).

In the chronic spinal cat cutaneous noxious stimulation may produce long-lasting inhibition of activity in CVC neurons supplying the paw and excitation of MVC and sudomotor neurons. The inhibition in CVC neurons is followed by an increase of blood flow through the skin and, consequently, to a long-lasting increase of temperature on the surface of the skin (Fig. 11 A). This inhibitory reflex has, as in animals with an intact neuraxis, a very distinct spatial organization: noxious stimulation of the skin of the contralateral extremity has either no or only a weak effect (compare Fig. 10 A with Fig. 11 A). The activation of the sudomotor neurons by noxious cutaneous stimulation is followed by an enhancement of the "ongoing" activity in these neurons (Fig. 11 B) which may last for up to 10 min following a stimulus of 10 s duration. The long-lasting inhibition of cutaneous vasoconstrictor activity and long-lasting enhancement of sudomotor activity can only be elicited by noxious cutaneous and not by innoxious cutaneous stimuli (compare Fig. 11 B and C). Thus, both depend on neuronal long-term mechanisms in the isolated spinal cord which are linked to the nociceptive input [20, 24]. It is unknown whether these types of exaggerated reflexes also exist in chronic tetra- or paraplegic patients; up to the present, they have not been described [44].

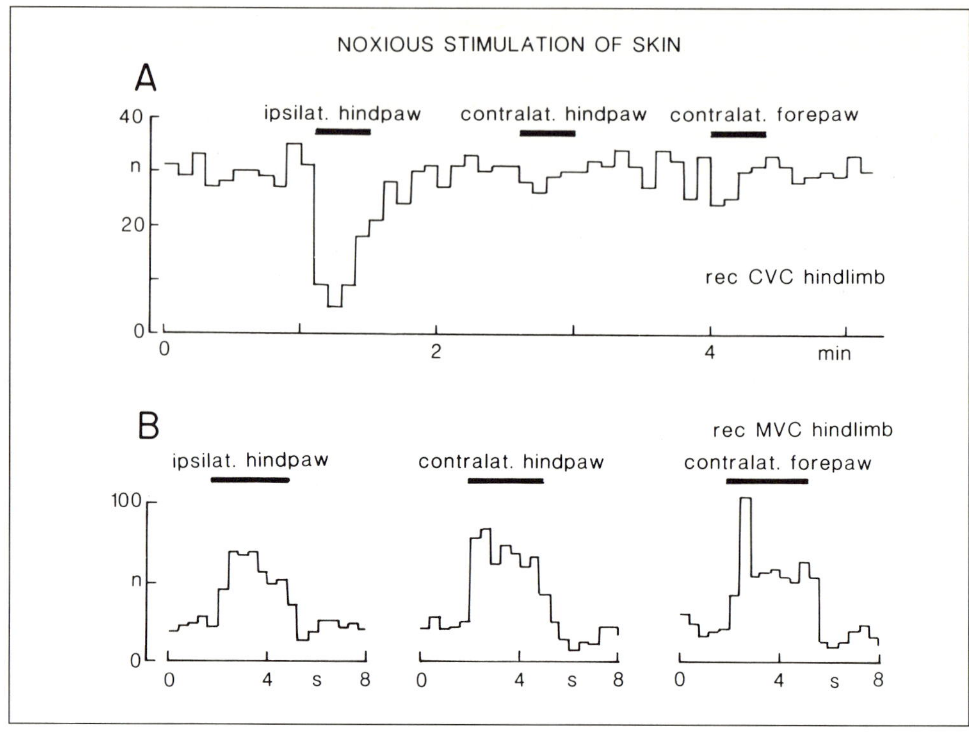

Fig. 10. Reactions of cutaneous vasoconstrictor (CVC) neurons (A) and muscle vasoconstrictor (MVC) neurons (B) to mechanical noxious stimulation (black bars) of skin in the cat. Note the spatial organization of the inhibitory reflex in the CVC neurons and the absence of the spatial organization for the MVC neurons. A, activity in two postganglionic CVC neurons; ordinate scale, impulses per 10 s (n). B Multiunit bundle (MVC); ordinate scale impulses per 0.4 s (10 times superimposed). (A) Jänig, unpublished; B) modified from Jänig, 1985)

These results strongly argue that the inhibitory reflexes elicited by noxious cutaneous stimulation are organized on the level of the spinal cord. The spatial organization of these reflexes indicates that the neuronal "reflex circuits" in the spinal cord are also spatially organized. It may be speculated whether these and similar yet unknown inhibitory spinal reflex circuits are activated by repetitive spinal cord stimulation leading in this way to decrease of activity in the vasoconstrictor neurons and, consequently, to an increase of blood flow through skin and deep somatic tissues.

Sympathetic outflow to the vascular beds is likely to be involved

In which way is the sympathetic outflow involved in the increase of blood flow through the diseased extremities during spinal cord stimulation? Answers to this question are speculative, given the present state of knowledge. The following points have to be considered:

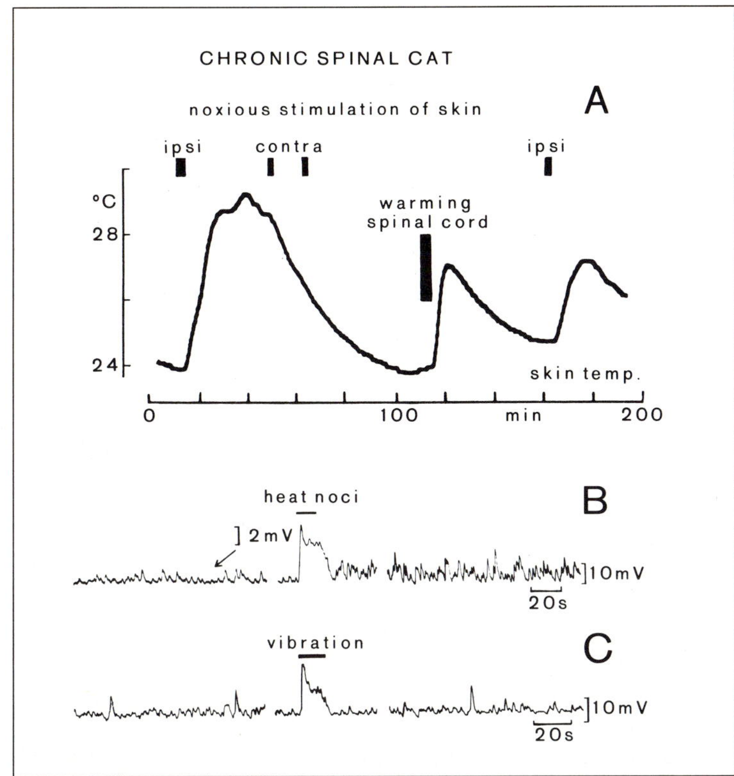

Fig. 11. Effect of noxious stimulation of skin on cutaneous vasoconstrictor activity and sudomotor (SM) activity to the hindfoot of chronic spinal cats (spinal cord transected between segments T_8 and T_{11} 108 days (A) and 72 days (B) before the experiments). A. Measurement of the temperature on the surface of the hairless skin of the left hindpaw. Note the increase of skin temperature (descrease of vasoconstrictor activity) upon ipsilateral noxious stimulation and upon warming of the spinal cord and its absence upon contralateral noxious stimulation. B, C. Recording of the skin potential from the hairless skin of a hindpaw (direct current, DC, recording) as indicator of the sudomotor (SM) activity. Note the increased SM activity following the noxious reflex (B), but no increase of SM activity following a reflex produced by non-noxious stimulation of skin (C; vibration, stimulation of Pacinian corpuscles in the paw). (A) Modified from Jänig and Kümmel, 1981; B) modified from Jänig and Spilok, 1978)

1) Vasoconstrictor neurons to skin, skeletal muscle, and other tissues are involved. The simplest assumption is that spinal cord stimulation decreases the activity in these neurons and in this way, induces an increase in blood flow. However, it is also possible that the pattern of discharge in these neurons is changed (e.g., from bursting pattern into more continuous activity) which then generates a dilation of the blood vessels. If this is the case, one might expect that the reflex pattern in the vasoconstrictor neurons (see Fig. 7) is changed during spinal cord stimulation.

2) Sympathetic vasodilator neurons are involved. In this case, these neurons must be activated in order to generate a vasodilation. Our knowledge about sympathetic vasodilator neurons is rather poor [14, 17].

53

3) Are sympathetic pathways to distinct sections of the vascular bed specifically involved? This would either require that different sections of the vascular bed are
   differentially innervated or that they are, as a consequence of the pathophysiological processes, differentially reinnervated.
4) Is the increase in blood flow induced by spinal cord stimulation related to other
   than the vascular effects of the sympathetic outflow? Does activation of sympathetic neurons induce neogenesis of blood vessels?
5) Finally, it must be kept in mind that the increase in blood flow occurs in ter-
   ritories which are already pathologically changed as a consequence of the
   peripheral vascular disease. As already mentioned above, it is well possible that
   afferent and efferent fibers which innervate the ischemic extremity undergo
   degeneration and regeneration. Under this condition the vasoconstrictor effect of
   impulse activity in vasoconstrictor neurons may be much stronger than in healthy
   tissue, and a small decrease of impulse activity may generate a large increase in
   blood flow. Finally, small diameter afferent fibers may no longer be able to dilate
   the microvascular bed under these pathophysiological conditions (see Fig. 3).

Experimental investigation of the mechanisms operating
during spinal cord stimulation: an idea

Spinal cord stimulation may lead to improvement of the nutritional blood flow
through the different compartments of the extremity, with relief of pain, disappearance of trophic changes, and healing of ulcera in patients with peripheral vascular disease. The mechanisms behind these effects are unknown. In order to establish
a more rational scientific basis of this therapeutic approach and to improve it,
systematic investigations of the patients, experimental clinical reasearch, and
research on animal models is necessary (Table 2).

1) The success of any experimental approach using animal models is dependent on
   a quantitative analysis of the clinical observations. These data are necessary in

Table 2. Experimental approach to mechanisms leading to increase of blood flow, relief of pain,
disappearance of ulcera during spinal cord stimulation (SCS)

---

1) Quantitative analysis of clinical data
   - Pain and paraesthesias
   - Perfusion of different compartments
   - Trophic changes
   - Time-course of changes during SCS and during conservative therapy
   - Relation to staging of arterial occlusion and degree of neuropathy

2) Clinical research on patients using modern technology

3) Research in vivo on animal models
   - SCS, var. position and strength of SCS
   - Recording BF through skin, skeletal muscle and joint capsule (LDF) (and possibly other
     autonomic effector responses)
   - Recording of activity from cutaneous and muscle vasoconstrictor neurones (ongoing activity,
     reflex activity) and from afferents

---

order to focus the experimental work on the relevant questions. The clinical investigations must concentrate on the following points:

- Pain and paresthesias (ongoing and evoked) which are present in the patients with ischemia before and during SCS.
- The perfusion of different compartments of the diseased limb (such as skin, skeletal muscle, etc.) must be measured. Does the blood flow in the contralateral, still sufficiently perfused lower extremity also increase during SCS? Does SCS stimulation perhaps also work in healthy extremities? An answer to these questions is extremely important for the design of the in vivo experiments on animals.
- The time course of the changes which are observed during SCS (separately for pain, paresthesias, blood flow changes, etc.) must be measured and compared with the time course of the changes induced by conservative therapeutic strategies. To what extent is the increase in blood flow and the relief of pain dependent on permanent or intermittent SCS? What are the stimulation modalities in the different groups of patients?
- What is the correlation between the therapeutic success of SCS and the staging of the arterial occlusion and the degree of neuropathy?
- The degree of sensory autonomic neuropathy in these patients must be quantitatively evaluated and correlated with the therapeutic success of SCS. These investigations will answer the question as to whether SCS is successful in patients in whom the sympathetic postganglionic neurons are more or less damaged (e.g., in diabetes mellitus).

To reach this aim vascular surgeons have to collaborate with other disciplines (neurologists, anesthesiologists working in pain ambulances, angiologists, etc.) and have to apply modern methodology. Quantitative data from these clinical investigations, first, will lead to recommendations which define the groups of patients which will most likely benefit from SCS and those which will not, and, second, will give the background material for a focused research on patients and for the design of animal models.

2) More sophisticated research should be done on the patients using modern technology, in interaction with the research on animal models.

3) The research on animals is in principle straight-forward (Table 2 and Fig. 12), although not easy to perform. This research should concentrate on the following points:
- Use of anesthetized animals. All the vital parameters, such as blood pressure, respiration, body core temperature, etc., have to be rigorously controlled. It may turn out that the rat is not an appropriate animal because it is too small and because its sympathetic nervous system may be different in the central organization from that in larger animals (including humans). These experiments can be extended to unanesthetized animals (simulating in this way exactly the situation in patients!) in order to measure behavior and other parameters (e.g., change of skin temperature, etc.).
- Stimulation of the dorsal surface of the spinal cord. The position of the stimulation electrode and the stimulation parameters (frequency, strength, pukse duration) should be systematically varied.
- Blood flow through skin, skeletal muscle, and joint capsule should be recorded using the laser Doppler flowmeter (LDF). This has to be supplemented by

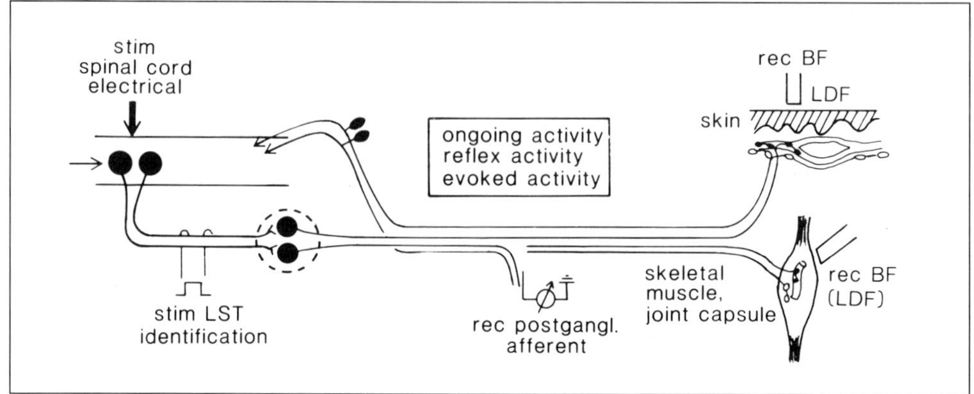

Fig. 12. Experimental design and set-up for studying the effect of spinal cord stimulation on activity in postganglionic vasoconstrictor neurons supplying skeletal muscle and skin and on blood flow through skin and skeletal muscle in animals. See also Table 2

     measurements of skin temperature (using a laser thermometer) and, if available, by thermography.
- Activity from sympathetic neurons innervating skin and skeletal muscle should be recorded directly in the anesthetized animals. Vasoconstrictor neurons can be recognized functionally. Changes of ongoing activity and its biological modulation during the cardiac and respiratory cycles and of controlled reflex activity by SCS has to be studied. These changes must be correlated with the changes in blood flow, etc. Antidromic activity which may occur in afferent fibers during SCS can also be recorded using the same neurophysiological approach. Results obtained in these types of experiments should give answers as far as the mechanisms which operate during SCS are concerned. This in turn may lead to new ideas to modify the therapeutic approach and the stimulation procedure.

Summary

In patients with peripheral vascular disease and ischemia of the lower extremities, electrical spinal cord stimulation may improve the nutritional blood flow, generate relief of pain, and alleviate trophic changes with healing of ulcera. In this way amputation as ultima ratio may be prevented. The mechanisms by which these positive therapeutic effects are brought about are barely understood. Most likely, they are related to the remote neural control of the small blood vessels of the ischemic extremity. Sympathetic neurons innervating these blood vessels are the most likely candidates. This article discusses 1) various aspects of this remote neural control, at the level of the effector organ and at the level of central integration in the spinal cord; 2) observations that argue that the beneficial therapeutic effect of spinal cord stimulation is related to the sympathetic vasomotor outflow to the affected extremity; and 3) strategies of clinical research on patients and research on animal models which aim to work out the mechanisms which are involved.

56

References

1. Bevan JA (1988) Basal tone in resistance arteries: role of wall stretch, flow and receptor specialization. In: Bevan JA, Majewski H, Maxwell RA, Story DF (eds) Vascular Neuroeffector Mechanisms, ICSU Symposium Series vol. 10, Oxford, Washington DC: IRL Press, pp. 1–14
2. Blumberg H, Wallin BG (1987) Direct evidence of neurally mediated vasodilation in hairy skin of the human foot. J Physiol 382:105–121
3. Boczek-Funcke A, Dembowsky K, Häbler HJ, Jänig W, McAllen R, Michaelis M (1992) Classification of preganglionic neurones projecting into the cat cervical sympathetic trunk. J Physiol 453:319–339
4. Brock JA, Cunnane TC (1992) Electrophysiology of neuroeffector transmission in smooth muscle. In: Burnstock G, Hoyle CHV (eds) Autonomic neuroeffector mechanisms, pp. 121–213, Harwood Academic Publishers, Chur, Switzerland
5. Chahl LA (1988) Antidromic vasodilatation and neurogenic inflammation. Pharmacol Ther 37:275–300
6. Chahl LA, Szolcsányi J, Lembeck F (1984) Antidromic vasodilation and neurogenic inflammation. Budapest: Akadémiai Kiadó
7. Esler M, Hasking IR, Willett IR, Leonard PW, Jennings GL (1985) Noradrenaline release and sympathetic nervous system activity. J Hypertens 3:117–129
8. Evans R, Suprenant A (1992) Vasoconstriction of guinea-pig submucosal arterioles following sympathetic nerve stimulation is mediated by the release of ATP. Brit J Pharmacol 106:242–249
9. Furchgott RF, Vanhoutte PM (1989) Endothelium-derived relaxing and contracting factors. Faseb J 3:2007–2018
10. Häbler H-J, Jänig W, Michaelis M (1984) Respiratory modulation in the activity of sympathetic neurones. Progress in Neurobiology (in press)
11. Hirst GDS (1989) Neuromuscular transmission in intramural blood vessels. In: Wood JD (ed) Handbook of Physiology, Section 6: Gastrointestinal System. Vol I Motility and Circulation. Bethesda, Maryland: American Physiological Society pp. 1635–1665
12. Hirst GDS, Bramich NJ, Edwards FR, Klemm M (1992) Transmission at autonomic neuroeffector junctions. Trends Neurosci 15:40–46
13. Hirst GDS, Edwards FR (1989) Sympathetic neuroeffector transmission in arteries and arterioles. Physiol Rev 69:546–604
14. Jänig W (1985) Organization of the lumbar sympathetic outflow of skeletal muscle and skin of the cat hindlimb and tail. Rev Physiol Biochem Pharmacol 102:119–213
15. Jänig W (1986) Spinal cord integration of visceral sensory systems and sympathetic nervous system reflexes. In: Cervero F, Morrison JFB (eds) "Visceral sensation", Progress in Brain Res 67:255–277
16. Jänig W (1988) Pre- and postganglionic vasoconstrictor neurons: differentiation, types, and discharge properties. Ann Rev Physiol 50:525–539
17. Jänig W (1990) Functions of the sympathetic innervation of the skin. In: Loewy A, Spyer KM (eds) Central Regulation of Autonomic Functions, Oxford University Press, pp. 334–348
18. Jänig W (1993) Vegetatives Nervensystem. In: Schmidt RF, Thews G (eds) Physiologie des Menschen, 25th edn, Springer, Berlin Heidelberg, pp. 349–389
19. Jänig W, Koltzenburg M (1991) Sympathetic reflex activity and neuroeffector transmission change after chronic nerve lesions. In: Bond MR, Charlton JE, Wolf CJ (eds) "Pain Research and Clinical Management" (Proceedings of the VIth World Congress on Pain), Vol. 3, pp. 365–371, Elsevier Publishers, Amsterdam
20. Jänig W, Kümmel H (1981) Organization of the sympathetic innervation supplying the hairless skin of the cat's paw. Journal of the Autonomic Nervous System 3:215–230
21. Jänig W, Lisney SJW (1989) Small diameter myelinated afferents produce vasodilation but not plasma extravasation in rat skin. J Physiol 415:477–486
22. Jänig W, McLachlan EM (1987) Organization of lumbar spinal outflow to distal colon and pelvic organs. Physiol Rev 67:1332–1404
23. Jänig W, McLachlan EM (1992) Characteristics of function-specific pathways in the sympathetic nervous system. Trends Neurosci 15:475–481

24. Jänig W, Spilok N (1978) Functional organization of the sympathetic innervation supplying the hairless skin of the hindpaws in chronic spinal cats. Pflügers Archiv 377:25−31
25. Jänig W, Sundlöf G, Wallin BG (1983) Discharge patterns of sympathetic neurons supplying skeletal muscle and skin in man and cat. Journal of the Autonomic Nervous System 7:239−256
26. Jobling P (1994) Electrophysiological events during neuroeffector transmission in the spleen of guinea pig and rat. J Physiol (in press)
27. Jobling P, McLachlan EM, Jänig W, Anderson CR (1992) Electrophysiological responses in the rat tail artery during reinnervation following lesions of the sympathetic supply. J Physiol 454:107−128
28. Johnson PC (1980) The myogenic response. In: Bohr DF, Somlyo AP, Sparks HV, Geiger SR (eds) Handbook of Physiology, Sect. 2, Vol 11. Bethesda: American Physiological Society, pp. 409−442
29. Lew MJ, Duling BR (1990) Arteriolar reactivity in vivo is influenced by an intramural diffusion barrier. Am J Physiol 259:H574−H581
30. Lew MJ, Rivers RJ, Duling BR (1989) Arteriolar smooth muscle responses are modulated by an intramural diffusion barrier. Am J Physiol 257:H10−H16
31. Linderoth B, Fedorcsak I, Meyerson BA (1989) Is vasodilatation following dorsal column stimulation mediated by antidromic activation of small diameter afferents? Acta Neurochirurgica, Suppl 46:99−101
32. Lisney SJW, Bharali LAM (1989) The axon reflex: an outdated idea or a valid hypothesis? News in Physiol Sci 4:45−48
33. Lovén C (1866) Über die Erweiterung von Arterien in Folge einer Nervenerregung. Berichte über die Verhandlungen der königlich-sächsischen Gesellschaft der Wissenschaft: Mathematisch-physikalische Classe 18:85−110
34. Luff SE, McLachlan EM (1989) Frequency of neuromuscular junctions on arteries of different dimensions in the rabbit, guinea pig and rat. Blood Vessels 26:95−106
35. Luff SE, McLachlan EM, Hirst GDS (1987) An ultrastructural analysis of the sympathetic neuromuscular junctions on arterioles of the submucosa of the guinea pig ileum. J comp Neurol 257:578−595
36. McLachlan EM, Jänig W (1983) The cell bodies of origin of sympathetic and sensory axons in some skin and muscle nerves of the cat's hindlimb. J comp Neurol 214:115−130
37. Mense S (1986) Slowly conducting afferent fibers from deep tissues: neurobiological properties and central nervous actions. Progress in Sensory Physiology, Vol 6, Springer-Verlag, Heidelberg Berlin, pp. 139−219
38. Mense S (1993) Nociception from skeletal muscle in relation to clinical pain. Pain 54:241−289
39. Morris JL, Gibbins IL (1992) Co-transmission and neuromodulation. In: Burnstock G, Hoyle CHV (eds) Autonomic neuroeffector mechanisms, pp. 33−119, Harwood Academic Publishers, Chur, Switzerland
40. Neild TO (1987) Actions of neuropeptide Y on innervated and denervated rat tail arteries. J Physiol 386:19−30
41. Rowell LB (1986) Human circulation. Regulation during physical stress. Oxford University Press, New York Oxford
42. Smiesko V, Johnson PC (1993) The arterial lumen is controlled by flow-related shear stress. News in Physiol Sci 8:34−38
43. Szolcsányi J (1988) Antidromic vasodilation and neurogenic inflammation. Agents Actions 23:4−11
44. Wallin G, Stjernberg L (1984) Sympathetic activity in man after spinal cord injury. Outflow to skin below the lesion. Brain 107:183−198

Author's address:

Prof. Dr. W. Jänig
Physiologisches Institut
Christian-Albrechts-Universität
Olshausenstr. 40
D-24098 Kiel
FRG

58

Neuropathic pain and stimulation of the nervous system

J. Gybels

Department of Neurosurgery, K. U. L. University of Leuven, Leuven, Belgium

Introduction

From a clinical point of view, two major categories of chronic pain have been recognized. One, often referred to as "somatic" or "nociceptive" pain, is hypothesized to be due to prolonged activity of these nociceptors whose activation also leads to acute pain. This is probably an important mechanism of pain in vascular disease. It is a common clinical observation that skeletal muscle pain is particularly severe during contraction under conditions of ischemia, and there are nociceptive fibers which are known to discharge maximally when a muscle contracts under ischemic conditions [8]. Ischemia of the muscles of the limb during exercise, ischemia of the skin, secondary changes such as ulcerations, and impairment of venous return are all factors which may intervene in the physiopathology of pain in vascular disease by activating different classes of nociceptors.

The other major category of chronic pain, often referred to as "central," "deafferentation," "dysaesthetic," "neuropathic" or "neurogenic" pain, results from injury in the nervous system. This pain does not depend on activation of nociceptors, but must be the result of changes in the signal elaborating machinery. Exactly where and how in the various subgroups of pain related to intrinsic neural abnormality the substrates of the pain sensation swing into activation remains, to a large extent, to be elucidated. It seems very probable that in advanced stages of an occlusive disease and in vasospastic syndromes neuropathic components may be an element of the pain-producing mechanism; ischemia of the nerve may indeed lead to a lesion of the nerve fibers and hence to neuropathic pain.

A few definitions

This deafferentation, neuropathic, central pain is characterized by some symptoms and signs for which the International Association for the Study of Pain (IASP) has given the following definitions [9] (this list is not complete):

1) *Allodynia*: Pain due to a stimulus which does not normally provoke pain.
2) *Analgesia*: Absence of pain in response to stimulation which would normally be painful.
3) *Anaesthesia dolorosa*: Pain in an area or region which is anaesthetic.
4) *Causalgia:* A syndrome of sustained burning pain, allodynia, and hyperpathia after a traumatic nerve lesion, often combined with vasomotor and sudomotor dysfunction and later trophic changes.
5) *Dysaesthesia:* An unpleasant abnormal sensation, whether spontaneous or evoked.

59

6) *Hyperaesthesia:* Increased sensitivity to stimulation, excluding the special senses.
7) *Hyperalgesia:* An increased response to a stimulus which is normally painful.
8) *Hyperpathia:* A painful syndrome, characterized by increased reaction to a stimulus, especially a repetitive stimulus, as well as an increased threshold.
9) *Paraesthesia:* An abnormal sensation, whether spontaneous or evoked.

Some remarks on the physiopathology of neuropathic pain

In recent years substantial progress has been made in the physiopathology of neuropathic pain. This is a vast topic and only a few remarks are appropriate here. (There interested reader can find much information in [1, 2, 3, 11, 16]. We will only consider neuropathic pain due to pathology in the peripheral nerve and stress that, besides peripheral mechanisms, central factors have to be considered as well.

The complaints that patients with neuropathic pain report is much more than just the presence of pain; they describe, for example, allodynia, a continuous, often burning sensation and flashes of excruciating, stabbing pain. Obviously, the diseases which are considered here start in the periphery, and several peripheral mechanisms which may be instrumental in the genesis of the different clinical characteristics of these pains have been clearly identified. Between these peripheral mechanisms one can cite as examples ectopic impulse generation, cross-talk between nerve fibers and increased mechanoreceptive sensitivity of afferent nerve fibers. Besides these peripheral mechanisms, mechanisms operating in the central nervous system have also to be considered (for discussion see [15]). Between the many arguments in favor of a central component in the physiopathology of these pains a striking argument is the observation that excluding the peripheral nerve proximal to the lesion, either by local anesthesia or cutting the nerve, does not necessarily abolish the pain. A well-known study in this respect is the one in which Noordenbos and Wall [12] described the failure of nerve resection and grafting to cure chronic pain produced by nerve lesions. These patients had the site of the original partial nerve damage reconstructed by total nerve resection of the damaged area followed by cable grafting of the sural nerve across the gap of the excised nerve. All seven patients successfully generated their nerves across the graft but the pain returned in the precise state and location of the pain they had experienced before the graft. It is to be observed that in these patients the sural lesions produced no painful sequelae and that although the whole nerve in which the original trauma had taken place was cut before grafting the painful symptoms returned only in that fraction of the nerve's territory involved in the original trauma.

Separate classes of central mechanisms such as, for example, central changes generated by instability of central control mechanisms, biochemical changes generated by the absence or the presence of substances transported from the periphery centrally, etc., have been hypothesized and are now the subject of intense scrutiny. The therapeutic implication is that it will be necessary to develop strategies aimed at diagnosing and correcting not "pain", but the different elements which in a given patient are operating and conditioning his/her pain experience.

Table 1. Pain Syndromes most likely to respond to SCS

---

1. Lesions of peripheral nerve and roots
   - Post-traumatic neuropathy
   - Low back pain with radicular pain due to arachnoiditis and epidural fibrosis, mostly after failed back surgery
   - Post-amputation stump and phantom pain
   - Post-herpetic and diabetic neuropathy
   - Partial plexus lesions caused by trauma, cancer invasion and radiation
   - Causalgia and reflex sympathetic dystrophy
   - Cervical syndromes with radiculopathy
2. Lesions of the spinal cord
   - Paraplegia (radicular pain at the level of the lesion and pain below the lesion when sensibility is preserved)
   - M. S.
3. Peripheral vascular disease
   - Atherosclerosis
   - Diabetes mellitus
   - Morbus Buerger
   - Morbus Raynaud
   - Sclerodermia

Modified from Meyerson [10]

Specific indications for SCS

Neurosurgeons became really interested in neurostimulation for the treatment of "intractable pain" in the late 1960s. The immediate reason for this was the formulation of the gate control theory [7] followed by Reynolds' discovery [14] that electrical stimulation could provoke profound analgesia. Since then, neurostimulation has been performed at the level of the peripheral nerve (PNS), the spinal cord (SCS), the dorsal column (DCS), the brainstem and the thalamus (DB (deep brain) S), and the motor cortex (MCS). The interested reader can find and in-depth review in Gybels and Sweet [3].

Since in vascular insufficiency the posterior part of the spinal cord is the target for stimulation, we will limit our remarks to SCS. Over the years, with clinical experience, several pain syndromes have been identified which are most likely to respond to SCS. They are listed in Table 1.

Table 2 summarizes some results of SCS in neurogenic low back and limb ischemia collected after an extensive search of the literature for a monograph on the Neurosurgical Treatment of Persistent Pain [3].

North [13], in a recent review, compiled 45 clinical studies, representing over 2500 patients, and reported the percentage of success (defined as patients with at least a 50% pain relief) of SCS for each of these studies. The mean percent of success calculated from these studies is 54%. From a study now in progess, which evaluates the results of SCS in the 80 patients with neurogenic pain (failed back surgery included) implanted in Belgium in 1989 and from which 70 patients were available for long-term follow-up, it appears that the result of SCS was judged as very good to good by 52% of the patients. The interest of this study lies in the fact that the survey was conducted by an unusual independent third party, namly, the Belgian health authori-

Table 2. Results of SCS in neurogenic, low-back, and limb ischemia
pain

	N	% Success
Amputation/phantom limb	103	33
Brachial plexus avulsion	20	20
Paraplegic pain	21	33
Post-cordotomy pain	19	58
Spinal cord/peripheral nerve	21	38
Post-herpetic neuralgia	8	25
Low-back pain	487	58
Severe limb ischemia	21	71

ties who, under specific conditions, finance the reimbursement for the stimulation device (to be published).

Inspection of the clinical data of Table 1 gives some hints with respect to the working mechanism of SCS. With the exception of the category of peripheral vascular disease, pain syndromes which are categorized as nociceptive pain are not likely to respond to SCS. It is also known that for SCS to be successful an obligatory condition is that the stimulation evokes paresthesia which must cover the painful area. This may explain why phantom pain in paraplegia is not responsive to SCS, but may respond to stimulation of the somatosensory VPL nucleus where fibers from the dorsal column of the medulla carrying information to the sensory cortex make a synaptic connection with thalamocortical fibers. Since in many cases of ischemic pain there is no lesion of the peripheral nerve, and other categories of nociceptive pain do not well respond to SCS, there is reason to believe that in pain alleviation of peripheral vascular origin by SCS a specific mechanism must be operating. This has been extensively discussed and studied in animals by Linderoth and his colleagues [5, 6], who are of the opinion that SCS produces a segmental, transitory inhibition of sympathetically dependent vasoconstriction in peripheral tissue. In this respect, it is perhaps not without interest that in the clinical situation the suppression of ischemic pain with SCS is often accompanied by a feeling of warmth in the corresponding area.

In sharp contrast to the huge amount of animal investigations of stimulation produced analgesia in acute pain stands the paucity of experimental data on neurostimulation in animal models of persistent pain. It represents a typical example where clinics precede basic science. One such study has recently examined the effect of VPL stimulation in an animal model of neuropathic pain [4]. In this study, stimulation electrodes were implanted in the aimed for somatotopic area by means of thalamic evoked potentials. The results of this study show that mechanical allodynia, induced by partly ligating the rat sciatic nerve, could be abolished by VPL stimulation. Naloxone did not antagonize the effect of stimulation, suggesting that the observed analgesia is mediated by a non-opioid mechanism. It was also shown that VPL stimulation had no effect in sham-operated animals. Experiments of this kind are important not only because they allow to study mechanisms of action, but also because they may help to convince those who favor a placebo effect to explain the clinical results of SCS as summarized in Table 2. Indeed, since in neurostimulation, as with other surgical interventions, no double blind studies are possible, a critical attitude is in order. This critical attitude implies that one takes into account all available data, even when direct comparisons between clinical and experimental data have to be made with caution.

Concluding remarks

Spinal cord stimulation for pain is frequently not a single and simple procedure, but is rather a time-consuming technique in which attention to detail is of prime importance. It is, as yet, not possible to correlate a particular pain condition with an expected success rate, but SCS is more effective effective for neuropathic than nociceptive origin and particularly effective for pain suppression in those patients in whom a vascular disorder is present. The reversibility of the method, the low rate of complications, better selection criteria, and improved devices and implantation techniques make the method very attractive as an alternative treatment, although one has to keep in mind that long-term success is of the order of 50%, at least according to our estimation from the literature and our own experience.

Major goals to be pursued remain to elucidate the exact neurophysiological mechanisms of stimulation-produced analgesia, particularly in persistent pain, and critical evaluation of the clinical results by the use of appropriate measurement. Both these tasks are difficult and time-consuming, but not impossible.

References

1. Besson JM, Guilbaud G (1991) Lesions of primary afferent fibers as a tool for the study of clinical pain. Excerpta Medica, ICS 981, Amsterdam
2. Fields HL (1987) Pain, McGraw-Hill, New York
3. Gybels J, Sweet WH (1989) Neurosurgical treatment of persistent pain, Karger, Basel
4. Kupers RC, Gybels J (1993) Electrical stimulation of the ventroposterolateral thalamic nucleus (VPL) reduces mechanical allodynia in a rat model of neuropathic pain. Neurosci Lett 150:95–98
5. Linderoth B, Fedorcsak I, Meyerson BA (1991) Peripheral vasodilatation after spinal cord stimulation: Animal studies of putative effector mechanisms. Neurosurgery 28:187–195
6. Linderoth B, Gunasekera L, Meyerson BA (1991) Effects of sympathectomy on skin and muscle microcirculation during dorsal column stimulation: Animal studies. Neurosurgery 29:874–879
7. Melzack R, Wall PD (1965) Pain mechanisms: a new theory. Science 50:971–978
8. Mense S, Stahnke M (1983) Responses in muscle afferent fibres of slow conduction velocity to contractions and ischaemia in the cat. J Physiol (Lond) 342:383–397
9. Merskey H (1979) Pain terms. Pain 6:249–252
10. Meyerson BA (1990) Electric stimulation of the spinal cord and brain. In. Bonica JJ, Loeser JD, Chapman RC, Fordyce WE (eds) Advances in Pain Research and Therapy, Vol 5. Raven Press, New York, pp 495–534
11. Nashold BS, Ovelmen-Levitt J (1991) Deafferentation pain syndromes. Pathophysiology and treatment. Raven Press, New York
12. Noordenbos W, Wall PD (1981) Implications of the failure of nerve resection and graft to cure chronic pain produced by nerve lesions. J Neurol Neurosurg Psychiat 44:1068–1073
13. North RB (1993) The role of spinal cord stimulation in contemporary pain management. APS Journal 2:91–99
14. Reynolds DV (1969) Surgery in the rat during electrical analgesia induced by focal brain stimulation. Science 164:444–445

15. Wall PD (1991) Neuropathic pain and injured nerve: Central mechanisms. Brit Med Bull 47:631−643
16. Willis W (1992) Hyperalgesia and Allodynia, Raven Press, New York

Author's address:

Prof. Dr. J. Gybels
Department of Neurosurgery
UZ Gasthuisberg
Herestraat 49
B-3000 Leuven
Belgium

Spinal cord stimulator: Design and function

K. R. Mullett, W. Starkebaum

Bakken Research Center, Maastricht, The Netherlands

Melzack and Wall published their gate control theory of pain in 1965 [8]. They proposed that small-fiber input associated with noxious (pain) information could be inhibited by large-fiber sensory activation. Pain perception depended upon the balance between large- and small-fiber input. They suggested that antidromic activation of the large diameter afferent fibers in the dorsal columns of the spinal cord could inhibit small-fiber input in the dorsal horns, thereby modulating the perception of pain.

Shealy and his colleagues implanted the first dorsal column stimulation system in 1967. Their report on the first series of six patients in 1970 established the feasibility of dorsal column stimulation as a means of modulating chronic pain [10]. Later, others demonstrated that pain suppression was particularly effective in ischemic pain and suggested that it was accompanied by or resulting from vasodilation of the peripheral microcirculation [1, 5, 7]. Linderoth concluded that this vasodilation resulted from inhibition of the sympathetic vasoconstrictor control [6].

The first dorsal column stimulating electrodes were placed subdurally over the dorsal columns by laminectomy. These early electrodes were of guarded bipolar configuration with a central cathode flanked by two anodes. The stimulating system consisted of an external transmitter which was inductively coupled to an implanted receiver. The radio frequency (RF) signal was transmitted across the skin where it was received and decoded by the receiver and then delivered to the dorsal columns by means of the lead system.

This early work demonstrated that stimulating the dorsal aspect of the spinal cord could be effective in modulating the perception of chronic pain. There were many problems with early stimulation systems [4] and many technical changes and improvements have occurred during the past 26 years. The three primary changes were:

1) Electrode placement was changed from subdural to epidural location in order to reduce the potential complications of spinal cord compression and cerebral spinal fluid (CSF) leakage.
2) Improved lead designs which allowed leads to be implanted percutaneously or by means of a small laminotomy.
3) The development of microelectronic circuits, lithium batteries, and hermetic electronic packaging have allowed for the design and manufacture of totally implantable stimulation systems.

These and numerous other design and technological innovations have led to the current state of design of Spinal Cord Stimulation (SCS) systems.

Design considerations

It is a fundamental assumption that dorsal column activation is essential either as a primary mechanism or as a marker of proper segmental inhibition for both the chronic pain and vascular disease applications of SCS. Electrode position is the most important factor in determining which axons in the dorsal columns are activated [9]. Theoretical modeling studies by Coburn [2, 3] and Struijk [11] show that other factors are also important including electrode polarity, electrode size and shape, electrode orientation and tissue impedance. The amount of cerebral spinal fluid between the dura and spinal cord is also an important factor since this fluid is relatively high in conductivity and tends to shunt current within the CSF and away from the spinal cord [11].

Surgical technique considerations are also important. Two main classes of SCS leads exist today – percutaneously and surgically implanted. Each has its own design opportunities and challenges. Stimulators must allow for non-invasive adjustments of stimulation parameters. Batteries must provide a sufficient capacity to meet the high current drain demands of the modality.

Spinal cord stimulation leads

SCS leads have four key elements: electrodes, conductors, insulation, connectors. They can be configured for percutaneous placement through an epidural needle or

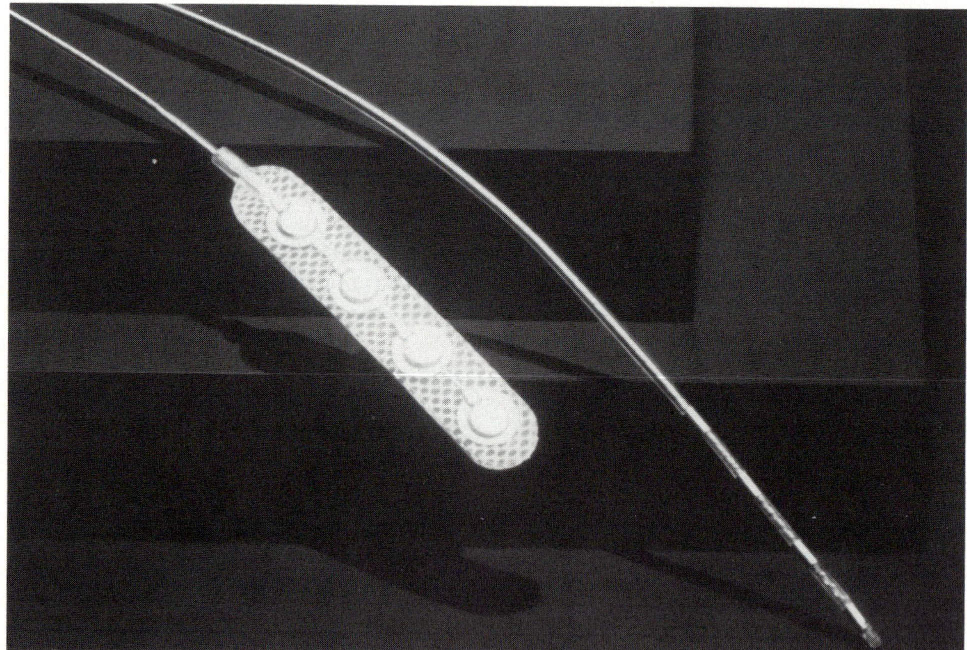

Fig. 1. Two types of spinal cord stimulating leads. The surgically implanted lead (left) is placed by direct vision through a small laminotomy. The percutaneously inserted lead (right) is placed through a Tuohy epidural needle

for placement with an open surgical procedure (Fig. 1). Either design must allow for placement under local anesthesia to allow the patient to cooperate with the surgeon in assuring that proper paresthesias are achieved in the affected part of the body.

Electrodes

SCS leads typically have from four to eight stimulating electrodes. They are usually fabricated from platinum or platinum/iridium alloy. The shape and maximum size of the electrodes for a percutaneous lead are constrained by the surgical technique and instrumentation. They are usually circular bands which surround the lead body. Electrodes span a distance of one to two spinal segments, although larger arrays are possible. Close electrode spacing is used for focal pains and wide electrode spacing for more generalized pains.

Surgically implanted leads are not constrained by the size of the implanting needle. These electrodes are typically flat plates captured in an insulating backing. This allows for various geometric patterns of electrodes to configure the stimulation pattern to the specific patient need.

Conductors

The electrodes are connected to a wire conductor by means of a YAG laser weld. This provides for a high integrity metallurgical bond between the metals. The conductor is fabricated from a fine wire that is wound into a helix. The helix configuration has two advantages:

1) A low stress, flexible structure that can be designed for durability.
2) A central lumen which allows for a removable wire stylet which facilitates lead placement in the epidural space.

The coil is designed so that the mechanical stresses in the individual coil wires are low to avoid fatigue fracture. Bending and compression are the main modes of deformation and cause of fracture in leads. Diameter of the coil, wire diameter, number of wires in the coil, coil pitch and material characteristics all affect the wire stresses which may lead to material failure. The designer must balance the durability requirements against the electrical characteristics of the lead. Decreasing wire diameter will decrease susceptibility to fatigue failure, but it will increase electrical resistance. This leads to increased power requirements from the stimulator. As in most designs, some compromise must be reached which optimizes durability and power consumption.

The metal wire itself is a nickel cobalt alloy called MP35N. This material is chosen for a combination of properties including high mechanical strength, excellent corrosion resistance, demonstrated biocompatibility in a variety of implant applications and it is available in fine wire sizes. This versatile high strength material is used in a variety of applications ranging from aerospace fasteners to orthopedic implants to stimulating leads.

Some leads use fine stainless steel conductor wires instead of coils. These wires are multi-strand for improved durability and conductivity. These wires are usually used for surgically implanted leads where a removable positioning stylet is not required. These wires are more suitable for attachment to the various geometric arrays of surgically implanted leads.

Connectors

A connection system is necessary to facilitate intra-operative testing, post-operative screening and subsequent connection to the implanted stimulator. The lead usually contains bands or pins which are inserted into a mating connector. Set screws have been proven to be the most reliable method of securing the connection, but other innovative methods to reduce size are now in evaluation.

Insulators

Some means of insulating the conducting wires, connectors, and electrodes from each other and/or body tissue must be provided. Polyurethane, silicone rubber, and Teflon PTFE tubes, coatings and glues are used. Materials used in neurostimulators have been thoroughly evaluated for biological compatibility and most have long and successful histories of use in other implant applications such as cardiac pacing, orthopedics, and urology. The unique demand of neurostimulation leads is to provide multiple isolated circuits on a small, flexible, durable lead. Teflon coatings as thin as 0.15 microns are being used to achieve these design goals.

Neurostimulators

The purpose of the stimulator is to generate a stimulating signal that is delivered by the lead to the appropriate nervous tissue. The stimulus is typically in the form of square, charge balanced pulses. Typical parameter ranges for neurostimulators are shown in Table 1. Compared to cardiac pacing systems from which these systems evolved, the power requirements for neurostimulators are quite high, primarily due to the higher frequencies and demand time required.

There are two types of stimulators in use today, the fully implantable system and the radio frequency (RF) partially implantable system.

Table 1. Typical neurostimulation parameters

Parameter	Range
Amplitude	$0 - 10.5$ V
Pulse width	$30 - 1000\ \mu$ s
Rate	$2 - 200$ pps
Cycle ON	0.1 s $- 24$ h
Cycle OFF	0.1 s $- 24$ h
Electrode selectability	$4 - 8$ electrodes, each $+$, $-$, or OFF

Fully implantable stimulators

Power source

One of a family of lithium battery systems is used in implantable stimulators today. While most pacemakers use lithium iodide (Li/I_2) batteries, the lithium thionyl chloride ($LiSOCl_2$) system is best suited to the needs of the fully implantable neurostimulators because of its higher voltage and energy density (Table 2).

Table 2. Battery chemistry

	Cell voltage (Volts)	Energy density (Watt-hours/cm^3)
$LiSOCl_2$	3.7	1.12
LiI_2	2.8	0.76
$LiMO_2$	3.0	0.90

Electronic circuitry

The electronic circuitry is divided into digital and analog sections. The digital circuit contains all of the logic necessary to control the behavior of the device. The analog section generates and delivers the therapy pulses to the lead via the feedthroughs and connector on the device. Typical logic circuits may contain up to 10 000 or more transistors. Three micron technology is required to fabricate a 5-mm square circuit chip. Much of the circuit area is taken up by the switching transistors which are used to control the programming of the electrodes. The analog circuit requires five micron tracks and is of a similar size.

The digital and analog circuits and other components are mounted on a "hybrid" which utilizes a multi-layer ceramic substrate. A small antenna is used for receiving and transmitting signals between the stimulator and the external programmer.

Electronic packaging, feedthroughs, and connector

The hybrid circuit and battery are sealed in a hermetic (moisture proof) package to isolate the electronic circuitry and battery from the body environment. The package is composed of a titanium can whose halves are laser welded together in a dry nitrogen atmosphere at the time of final assembly. Feedthroughs are a critical part of the assembly. They conduct the therapy pulse from the hermetically sealed circuits to the connector block. The lead or extension is secured in the connector with setscrews that are sealed by grommets to prevent stimulation at the connector site and corrosion of the connector components. Silicone rubber sealing rings limit fluid leakage into the connection from the lead side.

The fully implantable system requires a programmer to non-invasively set the stimulation parameters. This programmer is a computer-like device with a key board, display, and a "programming head". The system may use a custom-designed or standard personal computer to communicate with the implanted stimulator.

The typical pulse generator is 10-mm thick with a volume of 23 cubic centimeters and weighs 49 grams. About two-thirds of the volume is taken by the battery and one-third by the electronic circuitry (Fig. 2). The battery should last 5 years with typical neurostimulation parameters.

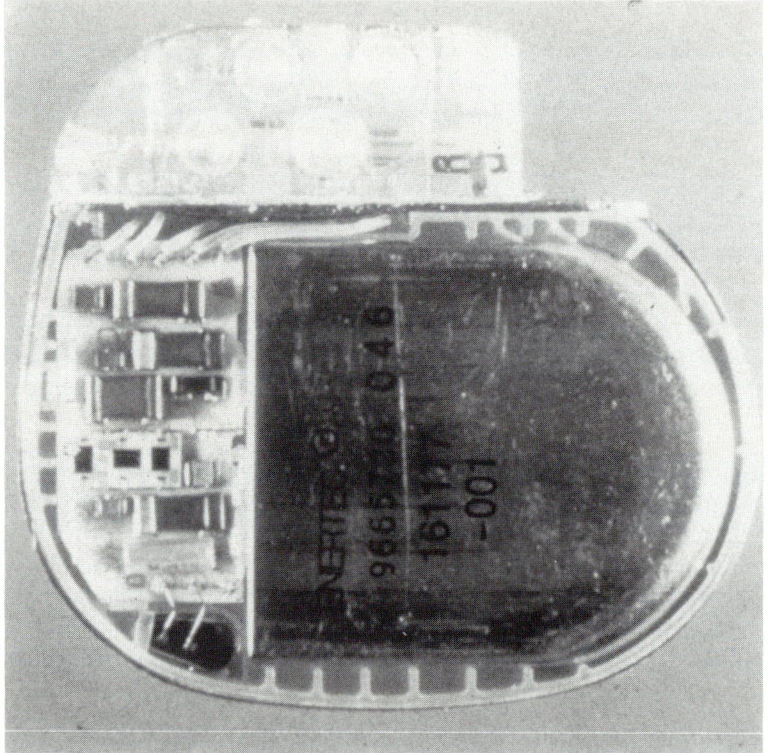

Fig. 2. The fully implanted neurostimulator consists of a lithium battery (right) and hybrid circuit (left) containing analog and digital circuit chips

Radio frequency stimulators

RF systems have the same basic elements as the fully implantable device, including a power source, electronic control and output circuits, packaging, and a programming system. These elements are divided between a passive implantable receiver that receives control signals and power for the therapy pulse from an external transmitter worn and operated by the patient (Fig. 3). The receiver has an antenna for receiving the signals from the transmitter. A hybrid circuit decodes the RF signal and delivers the therapy pulses to the receiver connector. Receivers are typically encapsulated in an inert polymer such as epoxy resin. This maximizes the efficiency of the RF signal which would be partially blocked if a metal package was used. The connector on the receiver is similar to the fully implantable system.

The transmitter is typically powered by 9-V or AA batteries. It contains all of the necessary patient and physician controls to define the therapy pulse. The output of the transmitter is coupled to the receiver by an antenna placed over the implanted receiver.

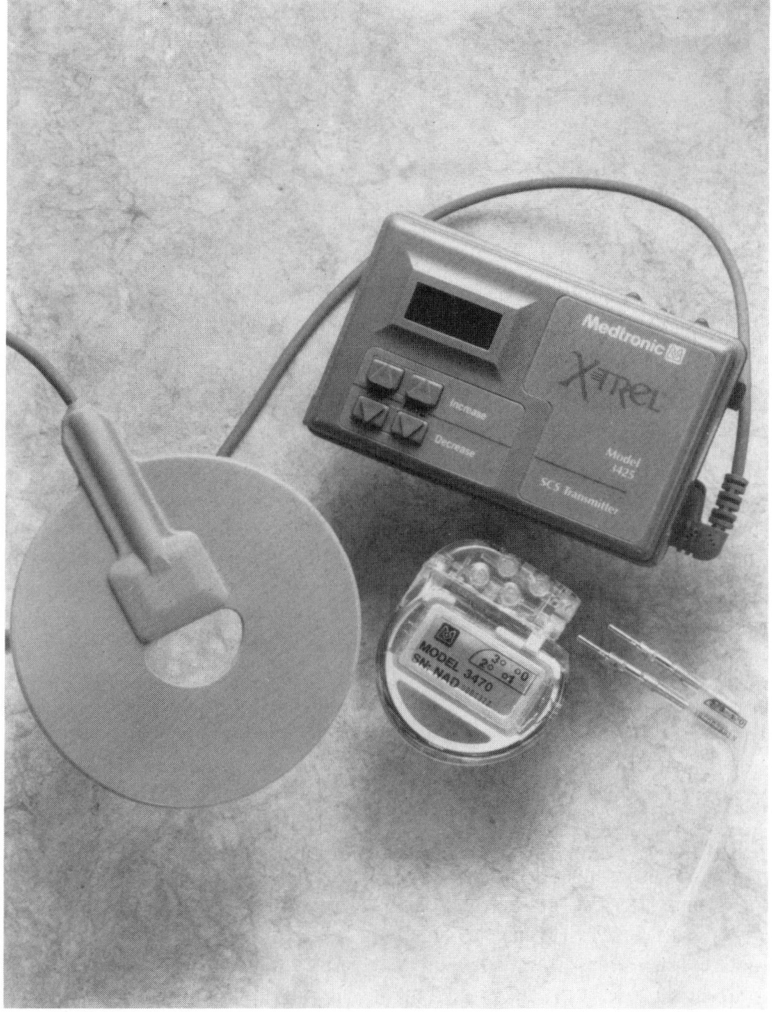

Fig. 3. A radio frequency stimulation system consists of the external transmitter (upper right), an antenna (left), an implanted receiver (right), and a lead system (lower right)

Summary

SCS systems are designed to provide the physician and patient with maximum flexibility and a variety of options. Stimulating leads can be percutaneously or surgically implanted. Percutaneously implanted leads are less invasive to implant and are best for focused stimulation because of their narrow electrodes. They may be difficult to place in a previously-operated, scarred back and may dislodge in active patients. Surgically implanted leads require a somewhat more invasive procedure, but have the advantage of being secured under direct vision in the epidural space. Their larger electrodes and varied geometries provide a broader stimulation pattern. They are often used when percutaneous implant is not technically possible (Table 3).

Fully implantable SCS systems are simple for the patient to use and require a minimum of patient involvement. They are more appealing cosmetically. Stimulation parameters are fully under the control of the physician. RF systems should be used when stimulation energy requirements are high, making the fully implantable system a poor economic choice. RF systems may be a better choice for patients who require frequent adjustments in their stimulation parameters (Table 4).

Table 3. Comparison of stimulating leads

Percutaneous	Surgical
less invasive	Secure placement
Focused stimulation	Broad stimulation

Table 4. Comparison of neurostimulators

Fully implantable	Radio frequency
simple for patient	low battery cost
Cosmetically appealing	More patient control
Physician controls parameters	

Future directions and considerations

Over the past two decades, SCS has evolved into an accepted and effective means of treatment of chronic pain and critical limb ischemia. Many technical challenges remain however. Diminished clinical efficacy due to lead migration is probably the most frequent complication. Improved leads and anchoring systems are required in the future. Electrode systems with more electrodes to allow recapture of paresthesia may also lead to improved results. More sophisticated electrode patterns may also be effective in directing the stimulus to more specific targets.

As systems become more complex and sophisticated, there is a continuing challenge to ensure that the systems are easy to use for both the physician and patient. This is particularly true of programmers and transmitters. There are probably opportunities to simplify surgical techniques as well. New and more complex fully implantable systems which extend the pulse repetition frequency and number of electrodes will create a demand for increased battery capability. Increased battery size and new battery chemistries may be required to ensure that the battery life is acceptable.

References

1. Augustinsson LE, Carlsson CA, Holm J, Jivegard L (1985) Epidural electrical stimulation in severe limb ischemia. Ann Surg 202:104–110
2. Coburn B, Sin W (1985) A theoretical study of epidural electrical stimulation of the spinal cord – part I: Finite element analysis of stimulus fields. IEEE Trans Biomed Eng 32:971–977
3. Coburn B (1985) A theoretical study of epidural electrical stimulation of the spinal cord – part II: Effects on long myelinated fibers. IEEE Trans Biomed Eng 32:978–986
4. Fox J (1974) Dorsal column stimulation for relief of intractable pain: problems encountered with neuropacemakers. Surg Neurol 2:59–64
5. Jacobs MJHM, Jörning PJG, Joshi SR, Kitslaar PJEHM, Slaaf DW, Reneman RS (1988) Epidural spinal cord electrical stimulation improves microvascular blood flow in severe limb ischemia. Ann Surg 207:179–183
6. Linderoth B, Fedorcsak I, Meyerson BA (1991) Peripheral vasodilatation after spinal cord stimulation: Animal studies of putative effector mechanisms. Neurosurgery 28:187–195
7. Meglio M, Cioni B, Dal Lago A, et al. (1981) Pain control and improvement of peripheral blood flow following epidural spinal cord stimulation: case report. J Neurosurg 54:821–823
8. Melzack R, Wall P (1965) Pain mechanisms: A new theory. Science 150:971–979
9. Mullett KR, Rise MT, Shatin D (1992) Design and function of spinal cord stimulators – theoretical and developmental considerations. Pain Digest 1:281–287
10. Shealy C, Mortimer J, Hagfors N (1970) Dorsal column electroanalgesia. J Neurosurg 32:560–564
11. Struijk J, Holsheimer J, van Veen BK et al. (1991) Epidural spinal cord stimulation: Calculation of field potentials with special reference to dorsal column nerve fibers. IEEE Trans Biomed Eng 38:104–110

Authors' address:

K.R. Mullett, M.S.E.E.
Bakken Research Center
Endepolsdomein 5
NL-6229 GW Maastricht
The Netherlands

Epidural spinal cord stimulation (ESCS): Implantation technique

K. Ktenidis, L. Claeys, S. Horsch

Academic Teaching Hospital Cologne-Porz, Department of Vascular Surgery

Introduction

Epidural spinal cord stimulation (ESCS) has been scientifically documented as a potent measure in the treatment of chronic pain for over 20 years [1]. The first ESCS application in the treatment of ischemic rest pain was in 1976 by Cook et al. [2]. Since 1986, we have studied the clinical effects of ESCS in patients with non-reconstructable peripheral arterial occlusive disease (PAOD) [3].

Indication for implantation

Apart from neurosurgical indications, one of the indications for spinal cord stimulation is critical ischemia of the extremities with rest pain and/or necrosis in patients with chronic peripheral arterial occlusive disease. In these cases the conservative procedures were unsuccessful and the vascular reconstruction or other operative vascular procedures are impossible or failed.

Furthermore, we see an indication in the following pain syndromes: phantom limb pain after amputation, Buerger's disease, Raynaud's syndrome, Sudeck's disease, scleroderma and other collagenosis with vascular establishment. Other indications may be therapy-resistent angina pectoris and impotence caused by vascular or neurogenous reasons.

Contraindication

The following conditions are considered contra-indications: pregnancy, drug addiction, chronic alcohol abuse, mental disease, incurable tumor, as well as severe diseases of heart, lungs of kidneys with short life expectancy.

Technical display

In addition to the usual operating equipment, an image converter control with a picture documentation facility, is required at the implantation.

The SCS system consists of a quadripolar electrode, an extension lead and a pulse generator. An external pulse generator is necessary for intraoperative and external trial stimulation.

The output of the pulse generator can be switched alternatively ON or OFF by briefly applying a control magnet. The device may be given to the patient.

Surgical procedures

Under local anaesthesia and with the patient lying in a prone position a vertical lumbar skin incision is made. For the complete implantation of SCS system (probe, extension lead, pulse generator) a change of body position is necessary. With adipose patients the more prone position is adequate for the complete SCS implantation (Fig. 1).

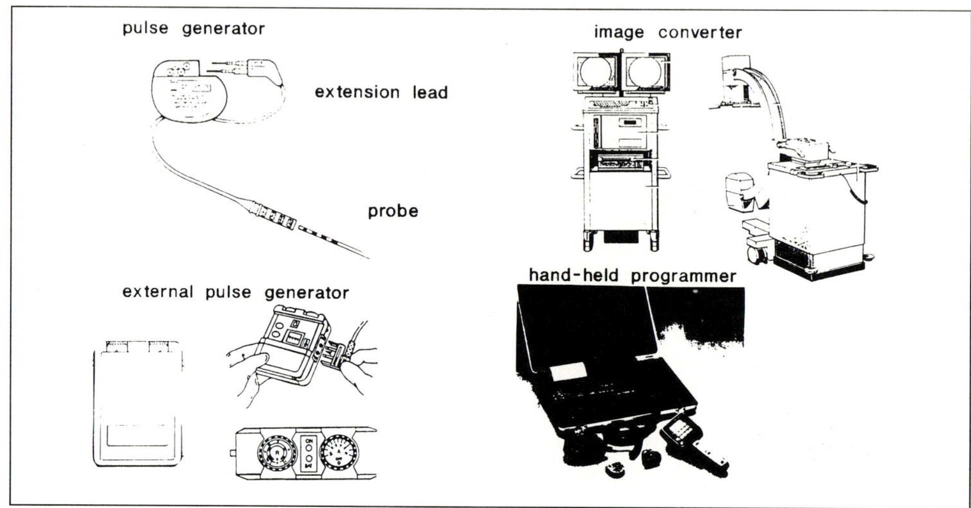

Fig. 1. Technical display

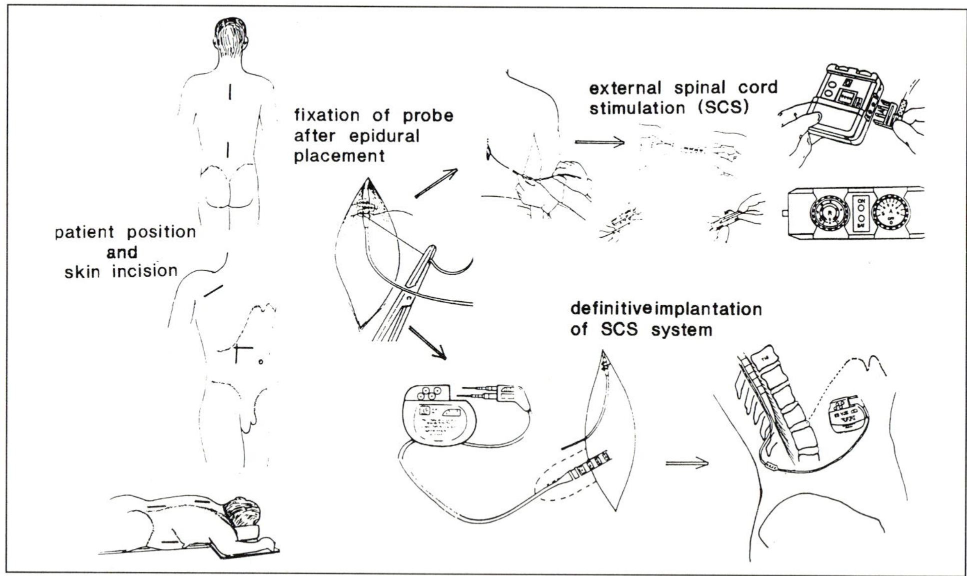

Fig. 2. Implantation of spinal cord stimulation

After denudation of the thoracolumbar fascia and palpation of the spinous process L3, L2 and L1 (or Th5, Th4 and Th3 for thoracic spinal cord stimulation), we perform the radiological imagery of the spine in anterior-posterior direction (Fig. 3).

Under x-ray control the puncture of the epidural space is performed with a special puncture needle (Tuohy needle). The angle of the puncture depends, apart from the anatomical condition, on the position of the patient on the operating table and the level of the puncture. Thus, the punctures on the thoracic level are, due to the physiological kyphosis, to be made flatter than lumbar punctures.

In order to achieve a standardization of the puncture, we position our patiens so that the physiological kyphosis or lordosis of the spine can be neutralized.

With the spinous and transverse process used as radio-anatomical (anterior-posterior direction) guide-structures, we now perform the epidural puncture adapted individually. The puncture on the exposed thoracolumbar fascia is performed 1−2 cm paramedian. Under image converter control (a.-p. direction) the needle during the puncture points to the spinous process above. Depending on the puncture level on the fascia thoracolumbalis, we distinguish between flat (level of spinous process) and steep puncture (level of transverse process). Figure 3 illustrates the exact performance of this procedure.

With lumbar puncture of the epidural space, we prefer the steep paramedian technique. The thoracal implantation of the SCS probe is usually performed above flat punctures. The puncture may also be performed in the midline (median puncture). Due to frequent breakage of electrodes, we avoid all median and flat paramedian lumbar puncture techniques.

In order to avoid the lesion of the dura mater the puncture is carried out according to the loss of resistance method. A further criterion for the correct position of the point of the Tuohy needle in the epidural area is the characteristic pierce of ligamentum flavum.

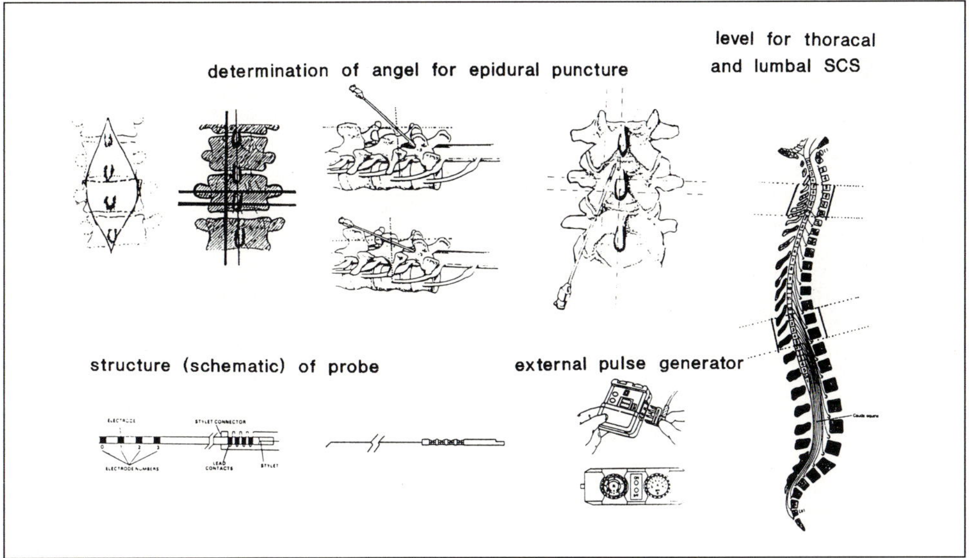

Fig. 3. Technique of the epidural puncture

For the lower extremities, the preferred puncture site is between the 2nd/3rd (or
1st/2nd) lumbar vertebrae. Under image converter control, the probe is pushed up-
wards epidurally to the thoracic 10th/11th level for stimulation of the lower extremities. The probe is located dorsally in the median line or above the dorsolateral
fasciculus of the clinical leading side (Fig. 3). The exact probe placement is performed under intraoperative stimulation, whereby pleasant paraesthesia occurs in
the affected extremities. For the thoracal spinal cord stimulation in cases of painful
diseases of the upper extremities, we insert the SCS probe between fourth and fith
thoracic vertebrae. The poles of electrode placed between C5/Th1. Initially, we carry
out a trial external stimulation. Indication for implanting a programmable generator
is provided when a sensation of warmth in the affected extremity occurs during this
stimulation, and significant pain relief is obtained.

The implantation of the complete SCS system may be performed in the course of
one operation on patients with intraoperative clear pleasant paraesthesia and warm
feeling in the extremities (Fig. 1).

The subcutaneously implanted generator can be programmed postoperatively and
transcutaneously by means of a portable computer. Permanent stimulation as well
as an intermittent circuit are possible. The frequency, amperage and current wave-
form can be externally altered by telemetry. The guidelines were $0.2 - 0.4$ msec for
pulse width, $80 - 120$ Hz for the frequency and $2 - 6$ V for the amplitude.

After-treatment

Apart from a low-dose heparin application, we usually prescribe a 24-h bedrest. Spinal cord stimulation starts at the first postoperative day. Under the prescribed
bedrest we first observe the spinal cord stimulation with the patient lying in supine
position.

EARLY POSTOPERATIVE PHASE

- Low-dose heparin application

- beginning of the electrical stimulation
  within 24 hours after implantation

- bed rest for 24 hours

- control of microcirculation (Doppler, tcpO2
  capillaroscopy) and quantification of pain
  reduction (analog scale)

LONG-TERM AFTER-CONTROL

- telemetric control of stimulation and
  possibly new programming of SCS generator

- control of the microcirculation parameters
  and of the rest pain reduction or the
  healing of skin ulcers

MEDIZINISCHER
IMPLANTATIONS-PASS
MEDICAL IMPLANTATION CARD

Patienten-Name
Patient-Name

Adresse
Address

PLZ Stadt
Zip Code City

Land   Tel.-Nr
Country   Phone No

System Modell-Nr
System Type No

Im Notfall Arzt benachrichtigen (siehe Rückseite)
For emergency please contact (see opposite side)

Im Notfall bitte benachrichtigen!

For emergency please contact.

Name
Name

Telefon-Nr
Phone No

Der Träger dieses Ausweises hat ein elektronisch
medizinisches Implantat.
The owner of this card is using an electronic medical implant.

Medtronic

Fig. 4. Postoperative care after SCS implantation

Postoperatively, we control the stimulation effect on the microcirculation (Doppler ultrasound, transcutaneous oxygen pressure, and capillaroscopy) and additionally register the rest pain reduction according to an analogue scale on a weekly basis.

For long-term control and possible telemetric reprogramming of the pulse generator, the patients visit the vascular outpatient department 1 and 3 months after discharge, and four times a year.

References

1. Shealy CN, Mortimer JT, Reswick JB (1967) Electrical inhibition of pain by stimulation of the dorsal columns: preliminary clinical report. Anest Analg 46:489–491
2. Cook AW, Oygar A, Baggenstos P, Kleriga E (1976) Vascular disease of extremities: electrical stimulation of spinal cord and posterior roots. New York State, J Med 76:366–368
3. Ktenidis K, Claeys L, Prudlo W, Requa U, Horsch S (1992) Role of the epidural cord stimulation in the severe ischemia of lower limbs. In: Progress in Angiology 1991, 7th European Congress of the International Union of Angiology, P. Balas (Editor) Edizioni Minerva Medica, Torino, pp 189–192

Authors' address:

K. Ktenidis, M. D.
Academic Teaching Hospital Cologne-Porz
Department of Vascular Surgery
Urbacher Weg 19
D-51149 Cologne-Porz
FRG

Definition, epidemiology, and pathophysiology
of critical limb ischemia

C. Diehm

Department of Internal Medicine and Angiology, Rehabilitation Clinic Karlsbad, FRG

> "Man is as old as his arteries and the arteries of men with critical leg ischaemia are very old. Treating such patients with severe leg ischaemia is unglamorous and ultimately a losing battle."
>
> *John Dormandy*

The evaluation and treatment of critical leg ischemia has been the concern of doctors from a wide range of traditional medical specialities that includes general and vascular surgery, angiology, diabetology, cardiology, hematology, and radiology, depending on both the local circumstances and national traditions.

Few problems in vascular medicine are as challenging as the management of critical limb ischemia (CLI), which may ultimately end in amputation and death. The author of this overview was a member of the working group that discussed and created a Consensus Document on Critical Limb Ischaemia. The basis for this paper is that document published in Circulation in 1991 [12, 29].

Definition of CLI

The earliest and most widely accepted classification of PAOD is that described by Fontaine et al. in the 1950s; he was, at that time, Head of the Department of Surgery in Strasbourg [13]. The Fontaine classification based on signs and symptoms has a long tradition and has clearly been found useful by many clinicians. The common meaning of the various stages involving severe ischemia is as follows:

Stage I

Patients in whom the condition is asymptomatic or oligosymptomatic, causing no or only mild and atypical discomfort in a foot or leg.

Stage II

Patients with intermittent claudication, where pain occurs after walking a certain distance and disappears at rest.

Stage III

Patients who complain of rest pain — severe persistent pain, usually localized in the forefoot, which is characteristically intensified when the limb is horizontal and eased by letting the foot hang down. Rest pain often prevents sleep and forces the patient to sleep in a sitting position. Strong analgesia is typically needed to relieve this pain.

Stage IV

Patients who have skin breakdown, causing ulceration or gangrene; it is generally associated with severe rest pain.

In the United States and United Kingdom the term *"Critical limb ischaemia"* is becoming more widely used than the corresponding Fontaine stages.

In 1982, Bell defined CLI as persistent and severe pain in the foot, at rest, preventing sleep and requiring repeated analgesia [3]. The symptom duration was greater than 4 weeks and superficial skin necroses of the foot or interdigital gangrene was required to make the diagnosis. Ankle systolic blood pressure measures were less than $40-60$ mmHg.

Both of the above definitions formed the basis for the discussion document from the First European Consensus Meeting on CLI in 1990 [12], now superseded by the Second European Consensus Document on Chronic Critical Leg Ischemia [29].

In this document critical limb ischemia in both diabetic and non-diabetic patients is defined by either of the following two criteria [29]:

Persistently recurring ischemic rest pain requiring regular adequate analgesia for more than 2 weeks
plus   an ankle systolic pressure ≤ 50 mmHg
and/or a toe systolic pressure ≤ 30 mmHg
or
Ulceration or gangrene of the foot or toes
plus   an ankle systolic pressure ≤ 50 mmHg
or   a toe systolic pressure ≤ 30 mmHg.

Critical limb ischemia is therefore ischemia which endangers the limb or part of the distal limb. Acute ischemia should be distinguished from chronic ischemia. Acute ischemia (e.g., that which results from an embolus) will not be discussed here, although it is recognized that for many patients with chronic ischemia there will be episodes of exacerbation, possibly caused by superimposed thrombosis.

A further recommendation was added in the Consensus Document for published reports or for the design and reporting for clinical trials. In addition to the above definition, further evidence of ischemia has to be obtained by angiography and/or one of the following tests:

– toe systolic blood pressure <30 mmHg
– transcutaneous oxygen pressure of the ischemic area ($tcPO_2$) ≤ 10 mmHg and which does not increase with inhalation of oxygen.

In diabetic patients sensory neuropathy alone can cause pain in the absence of ischemia. In these cases the toe systolic pressure measurements should be performed because a false high ankle systolic pressure is frequently found in diabetic patients due to Möckeberg's sclerosis of the media. A pressure of 30 mmHg is based on the fact that the majority of diabetic patients with a toe systolic pressure of less than 30 mmHg have a very poor prognosis [1].

Epidemiology

In comparison with coronary heart disease there is little information on the epidemiology of PAOD and especially of critical limb ischemia [9, 10, 33].

The true incidence of critical limb ischemia and amputations in the general population cannot be easily estimated. More is known about the incidence of amputation in the population of patients with intermittent claudication (Table 1). Two large epidemiological studies, the Framingham study and the Basle study, showed that only 1.6% and 1.8% of patients with claudication came to amputation [17, 27, 32]. The early hospital mortality following below-knee and above-knee amputations ranges from 3% to 10%. The hospital mortality after an above-knee amputation is nearer 20%. There are six series where longer-term mortality figures are quoted, ranging from 25–30% 2 years after amputation and 50–75% after 5 years [29].

Table 1. Epidemiology: Amputations statistics [29]

Incidence of major lower-limb amputations	Incidence*
UK district hospitals	120
Referral to UK limb-fitting centres	200
Veterans Administration (US)	260
Framingham Study (US)	300
Danish Hospital Survey	320

* million population/year
2nd European Consensus Document on Critical Leg Ischemia

In an extensive literature survey by Dormandy et al. it was found that even patients with claudication, but not critical ischemia, had a more than doubled mortality rate within 5 years, compared to the general population [9]. The life expectancy of the people affected is about 10 years shorter than that of a comparable control population.

From the studies referred to and from other data it can be estimated that the prevalence of peripheral arterial occlusive disease (PAOD) in the whole population is 5% in men aged over 50 years [14]. Progression of early stage PAOD to critical limb ischemia occurs in 20–30% of patients over a 6-year period and is estimated to affect 500–1000 patients per million adults [19].

For diabetic patients the incidence is higher; probably there is a five times higher risk for diabetics of developing critical leg ischemia. Ulcers and gangrene occur in 10% of elderly diabetic patients [18].

Concomitant Diseases

Several prospective epidemiological studies revealed that initially healthy persons developing PAOD had a four to six times higher morbidity from coronary heart disease compared with those remaining free of PAOD [5, 7, 16, 24, 27].

Up to 50% of patients with intermittent claudication and up to 90% of patients with critical limb ischemia have coronary heart disease [24]. The presence of PAOD also identifies a group of patients with high mortality from myocardial infarction. Therefore, it is now recommended that young and middle-aged patients with symptomatic PAOD, including those with critical limb ischemia, should be investigated by means of exercise ECG (if possible), echocardiography, thallium scanning, and coronary arteriography to identify those at high risk. CLI may be aggravated by emboli from the heart and other sites in some patients. It may more commonly result from the combination of arterial occlusive disease and decreased cardiac output, for example, from dysrhythmias, decreased myocardial contractility or drug-induced hypotension [20, 21].

Patients with PAOD are also at increased risk of cerebrovascular disease [16, 24]. The early-detected PAOD group in the Basle study developed signs of cerebrovascular disease three times more frequently than the controls. In PAOD patients, concomitant secondary hypertension due to renal artery stenosis is significantly more prevalent than in subjects without PAOD. Kidney disease caused by microangiopathy and/or pyelonephritis is particularly prevalent in the diabetic PAOD group. Patients with CLI are at a particularly high risk of arterial thromboembolism and, if bedridden for some time, venous thromboembolism.

Prognosis can be quantified by the rates of rehabilitation and mortality. In CLI rehabilitation is generally slow due to wound healing by secondary intention in 15% of the cases. A further 15% require re-amputation at a higher level, and frequently amputation of the other leg as well [30].

The fate of the patient with PAOD is, to a large extent, determined by the stage of the disease; even in the stage of intermittent claudication there is a threefold excess mortality mainly due to coronary heart disease and stroke.

Pathophysiology of CLI

In recent years, there has been increasing interest in the pathophysiology of critical limb ischemia because it is hoped that greater understanding of such disturbances may suggest new approaches to prevention and treatment, as much of our present treatment is still very empirical. Nevertheless, the pathophysiology of CLI in man remains to be established.

Pathophysiology of the macrocirculation

CLI occurs when stenosis or obstruction of one or more major arteries increases proximal limb vascular resistance so severely that the blood flow to the limb can no longer meet the nutritive requirements of the resting limb tissues.

Atherosclerosis is the underlying cause of PAOD in more than 90% of the cases, although inflammatory arteritis, which affects medium-sized arteries, or diabetic microangiopathy can also play a central role in this disease. In atherosclerosis, plaques form within the intima of the artery and there is proliferation of the cells in the vessel wall, accompanied by the formation of thrombi. These changes narrow the vessel lumen thus impeding blood flow and perfusion pressure to the more distal circulation, giving a reduced flow to the microcirculation. CLI occurs when arterial stenoses or occlusions impair blood flow to an extent where, despite compensatory mechanisms such as collateral formation, nutritive requirements of the microcirculation cannot be met. This usually results from the presence of multilevel disease or occlusion of critical collaterals.

Platelets and leucocytes (activated as they pass over ulcerated or ruptured atherosclerotic plaques or in poststenotic vortices) and impaired prostacyclin-like and fibrinolytic activity may promote arterial thrombosis.

Pathophysiology of the Microcirculation

The microcirculation comprises the arterioles, capillaries, venules, and initial lymphatic vessels. The importance of the microcirculation in critical limb ischemia is highlighted by the significant overlap between ankle/brachial pressure indices in patients with varying stages of PAOD. This overlap indicates that it is not just the macrocirculation that is responsible for the development of the signs and symptoms of PAOD and ultimately critical limb ischemia, but that changes in the distal microcirculation are of considerable importance in determining skin perfusion [34].

New techniques that have recently improved understanding of the skin microcirculation include capillaroscopy, fluorescence videomicroscopy [4] Laser-Doppler fluxmetry, and $tcPO_2$ measurements [15].

Combinations of these techniques give more information than any of the techniques used alone.

Compensatory responses to a reduced arterial blood flow include reflex dilatation and the development of a collateral circulation. However, the flow rate and the perfusion pressure in the distal circulation ultimately fall. This leads to claudication and later to rest pain and gangrene.

Although the exact sequence of events leading to reduced capillary perfusion in PAOD is unknown, mechanisms involved include the collapse of pre-capillary arterioles because of low transluminal pressure, arteriolar vasospasm, abnormal vasomotion, microthrombosis, collapse of capillaries due to interstitial edema, capillary occlusion by endothelial cell swelling, platelet aggregation, rigid adhesive leucocytes, rigid red cells or blood cell/platelet aggregates and local activation of the immune system. Fibrinogen levels are elevated in CLI, which further increases plasma viscosity and erythrocyte aggregation. Fibrinogen levels are increased by smoking, diabetes, and infection. The activation of platelets and leucocytes and damage of the vascular endothelium may result in vicious cycles between these cells via a range of mechanisms and mediators.

Skin microcirculation and disruption of normal vasomotion

Skin microvessels can be subdivided into thermoregulatory and nutritional vessels. Although the relative distribution of blood flow between the non-nutritional thermoregulatory vascular bed and the nutritional vessels varies considerably between different skin areas, nutritional capillaries usually carry less than 15% of total blood flow in the foot [4]. CLI occurs when a maldistribution of microcirculatory blood flow in the skin reduces the perfusion of the nutritive capillaries, which eventually leads to tissue necrosis (Fig. 1) [4, 29]. Total capillary blood flow is not the critical factor – in fact, in CLI total blood flow is often paradoxically increased because of arteriolar vasodilatation [22]. Therefore, the ultimate cause of CLI is presum-

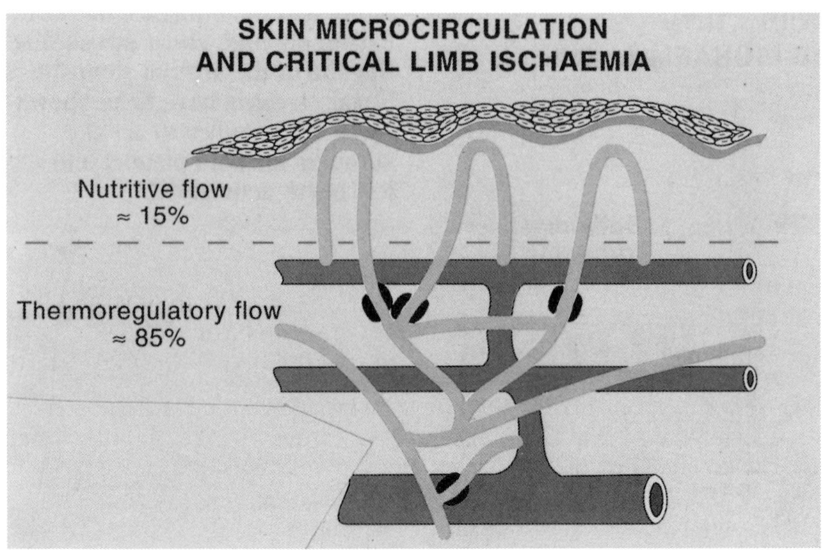

Fig. 1. Skin microcirculation and critical limb ischemia [8]

ably maldistribution of skin microcirculation in addition to reduced total blood flow.

There is also a circadian rhythm of blood flow to the foot, with the lowest values occurring at night, partly explaining why ischemic rest pain appears to worsen during night [2].

Vasomotion (low frequency waves of blood flow through the capillaries) is a normal phenomenon that occurs as the result of alternate constriction and relaxation of precapillary vessels. This vasomotion helps to distribute blood evenly throughout the microcirculation [31]. Laser-Doppler flowmetry of the skin has demonstrated an abnormal pattern on vasomotion in CLI [31]. In healthy limbs, vasomotion consists of low frequency waves of about three cycles per minute in the foot. In CLI, high-frequency flow waves of about 21 cycles per minute appear, which are only rarely seen in a normal limb. Loss of vasomotion may contribute to maldistribution of flow in the microcirculation, which causes underperfusion of some capillaries and no perfusion in others [29]. Interestingly, the pathological pattern of vasomotion can be corrected by percutaneous catheter procedures.

Impairment of blood rheology

In the healthy limb, the intrinsic flow properties of blood probably have minimal influence on blood flow through the microcirculation. Blood has a low viscosity, and normal erythrocytes are readily deformed by physiological shear stresses. Erthrocytes and leucocytes must deform to pass through nutritive capillaries, because their diameter is wider than that of the narrower capillaries. In the normal microcirculation they deform easily under high perfusion pressures and high shear stresses, even though leucocytes are much more rigid than erythrocytes [29].

88

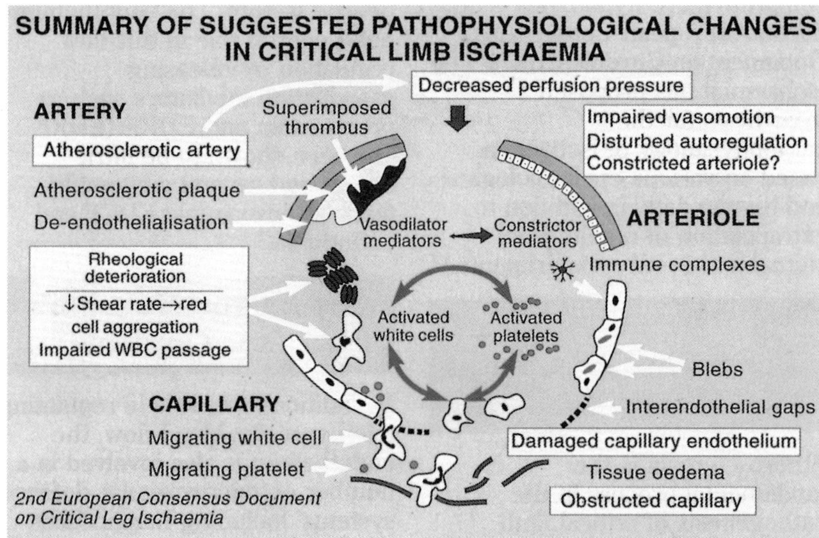

Fig. 2. Factors affecting blood rheology in critical leg ischemia [8]

The filterability of blood through micropore filters which mimic nutritive capillaries (pore diameter 5 μm) is decreased in PAOD, with a greater impairment in CLI than in patients with intermittent claudication. This impaired blood filterability in PAOD is thought to reflect the influence of the accompanying leucocytosis, hyperfibrinogenemia and increased plasma viscosity [8, 20, 21]. There is no apparent loss of erythrocyte deformability when filtration methods are used to assess leucocyte-free, washed erythrocytes from PAOD patients, where the influence of leucocytes and fibrinogen has been excluded.

In PAOD, blood viscosity increases due to an increased hematocrit and raised plasma fibrinogen level, changes that result partly from the influence of cigarette smoking. In critical limb ischemia, a further increase in fibrinogen due to ischemic necrosis, and occasionally infection, causes a more marked increase in plasma viscosity and erythrocyte aggregation. A reduced perfusion pressure and shear stress together cause a reduction in erythrocyte deformation and an increase in aggregation. An increased bulk viscosity then results from this decreased deformation and an increased erythrocyte aggregation [20, 21].

The additional consequences of ischemia such as acidosis, hyperosmolarity and calcium accumulation further impair erythrocyte deformability. It is likely that blood flow in the nutritive microcirculation is adversely affected by the changes in blood rheology seen in PAOD patients (Fig. 2).

Platelets in CLI

Peripheral arterial occlusive disease has been shown to cause a number of platelet abnormalities. A combination of both in vitro and in vivo studies using blood from PAOD patients has shown an increased turnover of platelets due to a shortened sur-

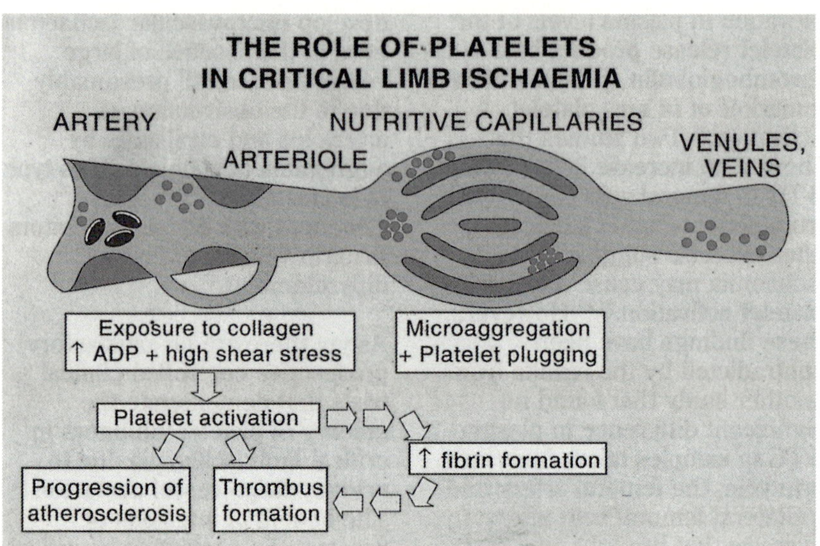

Fig. 3. The role of platelets in critical limb ischemia [8]

vival time, an increase in the mean platelet volume, a decreased platelet count, and increased platelet aggregation [6, 11, 20, 25, 28, 35].

Activated platelets express adhesion receptors and produce a variety of release products, which may promote vasoconstriction and fibrin formation and inhibit fibrinolysis (Fig. 3).

Abnormal activation of platelets is thought to be important in the pathogenesis of critical limb ischemia for a number of reasons. Activated platelets may encourage the progression of atherosclerosis by releasing platelet-derived growth factor (PDGF), which has been shown in vitro to stimulate smooth muscle cell proliferation. Activated platelets may aggravate tissue ischemia by releasing chemical mediators such as serotonin (5-HT) and thromboxane A_2 (TX A_2) which cause vasoconstriction of arteries. PAOD also causes a significant elevation in plasma levels of the platelet release product betathromboglobulin (β-TH), which is a marker of in vivo platelet activation.

Finally, the increase in platelet aggregation caused by PAOD is likely to be important in the pathogenesis of critical limb ischemia. Platelet aggregation in PAOD patients is accentuated by exercise that induces ischemia. Increased levels of platelet aggregates in the circulation correlate with the increase in plasma fibrinogen, seen in PAOD.

Fibrin formation plays a major role in arterial thrombosis. There are data showing that in toes of CLI patients up to 90% of 30 – 50 micrometer precapillary arterioles are occluded by microthrombi [29].

The role of leucocytes in critical limb ischemia

There is an increased evidence that white blood cells may play an important role in both the progression of atherosclerosis and in the pathogenesis of critical limb ischemia [20, 21, 26]. Patients with CLI have leucocyte activation, as shown by filtration studies, which is normalized after surgery. Leucocyte activation may occur as cells pass over an ulcerated atherosclerotic plaque, partly due to a chemical stimulus from contact with the damaged vessel lining and partly due to a physical stimulus of shear stresses at the site of the arterial stenosis. In vitro studies have demonstrated that leucocytes become activated when they are exposed to high shear forces. The presence of activated platelets has also been shown to activate neutrophil leucocytes.

The reduced filterability of activated leucocytes is likely to lead to plugging of nutritive capillaries within the microcirculation. Activated leucocytes also release a number of chemical mediators, including PAF, leukotrienes, superoxide anions, and proteolytic enzymes [23]. Leucocyte activation products have the combined effects of causing platelet aggregation, vasospasm and endothelial damage, all of which may contribute to the pathogenesis of critical limb ischemia. Thus, the leucocyte may be a possible therapeutic target for the treatment of CLI.

The role of the endothelium

PAOD causes a number of changes in the normal function of the endothelium, changes which are thought to be important in both the progression of atherosclerosis and the pathogenesis of critical limb ischemia. Elevated release of von Willebrand factor (vWF) has been reported in PAOD. This may promote platelet adhesion to the subendothelium and endothelium-derived constricting factor (EDGF) stimulating vasoconstriction. Hypoxic damage to the endothelium is thought to result in an imbalance in the secretion of EDRF and EDGF. A reduced production of EDRF allows leukotrienes released from activated leucocytes to provoke vasospasm, which further might exacerbate CLI [20, 21].

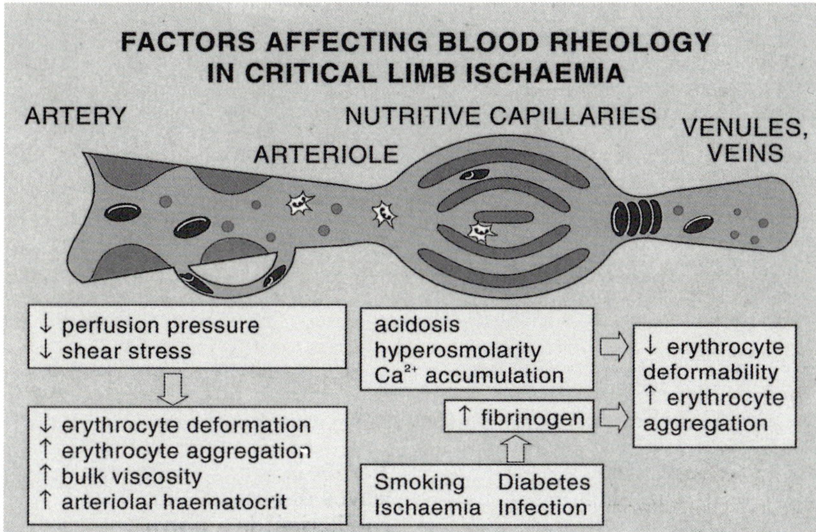

Fig. 4. Summary of suggested pathophysiological changes in critical leg ischemia at different levels of the circulation (WBC, White Blood Cell [29])

To summarize, the ultimate cause of critical limb ischemia is likely to be the maldistribution of blood to the skin microcirculation in addition to a reduction in total blood flow. The sequence of events leading to a decrease in the capillary perfusion is not yet established totally but several potential causes can presently be suggested [8]:

- collapse of precapillary arterioles because of low transmural pressure
- arterial vasospasm
- abnormal vasomotion
- microthrombosis
- collapse of capillaries due to interstitial oedema
- capillary occlusion by endothelial cell swelling, platelet aggregates, rigid and adhesive leucocytes or rigid red cells
- local activation of the immune system.

References

1. Apelquist J, Castenfors J, Larson J, Stenstrom A, Agardh CD (1989) Prognostic value of systolic ankle and toe pressure levels in outcome of diabetic foot ulcer. Diabetes Care 12:6, 115–120
2. Bartoli V, Dorigo B, Tedeschi E et al (1970) Circadian periodicity of calf blood flow in subjects with intermittent claudication. Angiology 21:215
3. Bell PRF (1982) The definition of critical ischemia of a limb. Working Party of the International Vascular Symposium. Br J Surg 69:52
4. Bollinger A, Fagrell B (1990) Clinical Capillaroscopy: A Guide to its Use in Clinical Research and Practice. Toronto, Hogrefe & Huber
5. Brothing S, Metelitsa VI, Barth W et al (1976) Prevalence of ischemic heart disease, arterial hypertension and intermittent claudication and distribution of risk factors among middle aged men in Moscow and Berlin. Cor et Vasa 18:104
6. Cella G, Zahavi J, de Haas HA et al (1979) Beta-thromboglobulin, platelet production time and platelet function in vascular disease. Br Haematol 43:127–136
7. Criqui MH, Coughlin SS, Fronek A (1985) Noninvasively diagnosed peripheral arterial disease as a predictor of mortality: results from a prospective study. Circulation 71:768
8. Critical Limb Ischemia. A Slide Lecture Kit (3), Lowe GDO (ed) Produced by professional Postgraduate Services, Europe Ltd, Worthing UK
9. Dormandy J, Mahir M, Ascady et al (1989) Fate of the patients with chronic leg ischemia. J Cardiovasc Surg 30:50–57
10. Dormandy JA, Stock G (eds) (1990) Critical Leg Ischemia – Its pathophysiology and Management. Berlin: Springer Verlag
11. Evans G, Irvine WT (1966) Long-term arterial graft patency in relation to platelet adhesiveness, biochemical factors and anticoagulant therapy. Lancet ii:353–355
12. First European Consensus Document on Critical Limb Ischemia (1990) In: Critical Leg Ischemia: Its Pathophysiology and Management. (Dormandy JA, Stock G, eds) Berlin: Springer Verlag, pp 1XXLV111
13. Fontaine R, Dubost C (1954) Les greffes vasculaires. Rapport au Congrès de Chirurgie, Paris, 226 ff
14. Fowkes FGR (1988) Epidemiology of atherosclerotic arterial disease in the lower limbs. Eur J Vasc Surg 2:283–291
15. Franzeck UK, Talke P, Bernstein EF, Golbranson FL, Fronek A (1982) Transcutaneous PO_2 measurements in health and peripheral arterial occlusive disease. Surgery 91:156–163
16. Hertzer NR, Raven EG, Young JR et al (1984) Coronary artery disease in peripheral vascular patients – a classification of 1000 coronary angiograms and results of surgical management. Ann Surg 199:223

17. Kannel WB, Skinner JJ, Schwartz MJ, Shurtleff D (1970) Intermittent claudication-incidence in the Framingham Study. Circulation XLI:875
18. Krolowski AS, Warram JH (1991) Epidemiology of diabetes mellitus, in Marble A, Krall LP, Bradley RS, Christlieb AR, Soulidner JS (eds) Joslin's Diabetes mellitus (ed 12) Philadelphia, Pa, Lea & Ferbiger, pp 12–42
19. Lasila R, Lepäntalo M, Lindfors O (1986) Peripheral arterial disease − natural outcome. Acta med Scand 220:295–298
20. Lowe GDO, Reavey MM, Johnston RV et al (1979) Increased platelet aggregates in vascular and nonvascular illness: correlation with plasma fibrinogen and effect of ancrod. Thromb Res 14:377–386
21. Lowe GDO (1990) Pathophysiology of critical limb ischaemia, in Dormandy J, Stock G (eds) Critical leg ischemia: its Pathophysiology and management. Berlin, Springer-Verlag, pp 17–30
22. Mc Ewan AL, Ledingham IMcA (1971) Blood flow characteristics and tissue nutrition in apparently ischemic feet. Br Med J iii:220
23. Mehta JL (1989) The role of leucocytes in critical limb ischemia. In: The Pathophysiology of Critical Limb Ischaemia and Pharmacological Intervention with a Stable Prostacyclin Analogue: RMS Services, pp 13–17
24. Müller-Bühl U, Diehm C, Sieben U et al (1987) Prävalenz and Risikofaktoren von peripher-arterieller Verschlußkrankheit und koronarer Herzkrankheit. Vasa, Suppl 21:1–53
25. Murphy EA, Mustard JF (1962) Coagulation tests and platelet economy in atherosclerotic and control subjects. Circulation 25:124–125
26. Nash GB, Thomas PRS, Dormandy JA (1969) Abnormal flow properties of white blood cells in patients with severe ischaemia of the leg. Br Med J 296:1699–1701
27. Nissen C, Schweizer W (1981) Koronare Herzkrankheit (1981) In: Basler Studie. (Widmer LK, Stähelin HB, Nissen C, da Silva A, eds) Bern: Hans Huber
28. O'Brien JR, Etherington MD, Jamieson S et al (1975) Blood changes in atherosclerosis after myocardial infarction and venous thrombosis. Thromb Diath Haem 34:483–497
29. Second European Consensus Document on Chronic Critical Leg Ischemia (1991) Circulation 84, 4:1–21
30. Stirnemann P, Nachbur B, Oesch A (1986) In: Angiologie 86 (Widmer LK, Zempf E (eds)) Berne: Hans Huber
31. Seifert H, Jaeger K, Bollinger A (1988) Analysis of flow motion by the laser-Doppler technique in patients with peripheral arterial occlusive disease. Int Microcirc Clin Exp 7:223–236
32. Widmer LK, Biland LDa, Silva A (1985) Risk profile and occlusive peripheral artery disease (OPAD), in Proceedings of the 13th International Congress of Angiology, Athens 9–14 June
33. Wolfe JHN (1986) Defining the outcome of critical ischemia: a one year prospective study. Brit J Surg 73:321
34. Yao JST (1970) Haemodynamic studies in peripheral arterial disease. Br J Surg 57:761–766
35. Zahavi J, Zahavi M (1975) Enhanced platelet release reaction, shortened platelet survival time, and increased platelet aggregation and plasma thromboxane B_2 in chronic obstructive arterial disease. Thromb Diath Haem 34:483–497

Author's address:

Prof. Dr. med. Curt Diehm
Department of Internal Medicine and Angiology
Rehabilitation Clinic Karlsbad
Affiliated Academic Hospital of the University of Heidelberg
D-76307 Karlsbad-Langensteinbach
FRG

Pharmacotherapy of critical limb ischaemia

J.F. Belch[1], P. McCollum[2]

University Departments of Medicine[1] and Surgery[2], Ninewells Hospital and
Medical School, Dundee, Scotland

Introduction

Peripheral arterial disease is a frequent cause of morbidity. Five percent of men in
the United Kingdom over the age of 50 years suffer from its most common symptom,
intermittent claudication [54]. Critical ischaemia which threatens limb survival develops in approximately 12% [58]. The second European Consensus Document on
critical limb ischaemia (CLI) [37] describes clinical CLI as patients who have persistent recurring rest pain requiring regular analgesia for greater than 2 weeks and/or
ulceration or gangrene of the foot or toes. An ankle systolic pressure of $>50\,mmHg$
is a further, though debated, requirement. A fundamental process in the pathogenesis of CLI is the development of atherosclerosis causing narrowing or occlusion of
proximal blood vessels which reduces blood flow and perfusion pressure to the distal
circulation. This is the primary problem in CLI which leads to the changes in the
microcirculation described below.

General considerations

Patients will frequently present with severe pain alone or in combination with ulceration or gangrene. The pain is difficult to control and usually requires treatment with
strong analgesics, often opiates in the form of morphine. The pain is worsened by
elevation of the leg and dependency only briefly improves the situation due to the
subsequent development of oedema which further impairs the already threatened circulation. Whilst one must be aware of the potential haemoconcentrating effects of
diuretic therapy, with a subsequent increase in blood viscosity, judicious use of such
therapy for the oedematous limb can relieve the tissue pressure and provide some
relief from the ischaemia. This is particularly so in the diabetic patient.
  The preferred treatment of CLI is surgical revascularization which will depend on
the anatomical level of the problem. Angiography should be the first step and
although probably less than 25% of patients have arterial lesions suitable for
angioplasty, this possibility should be assessed first [14]. In some of the frail or elderly patients angioplasty can be a first line approach. In the majority of cases, however,
surgical revascularization is appropriate and the short-term outcomes for surgery are
good with an 80% limb salvage in chronic CLI, compared to a mortality of 4% [35].
If the onset of CLI is acute, however, mortality and morbidity are greater. The death
rate is then around 25% and the change of salvaging the limb greatly dependent on
whether the occlusion is embolic, where the success rate is approximately 85%, or
thrombotic when the success rate falls to 50% [35]. The decision to treat by surgery,
angioplasty or pharmacotherapy is, however, often not an easy one. It primarily de-

pends on patient and disease-related factors but also on external factors such as local hospital facilities and the expertise of the various clinicians. Whilst a surgical approach must be considered the optimum treatment, as many as 1 in 5 patients with CLI may be unsuitable for surgery for a variety of reasons [55].

A plethora of drugs is marketed as being useful in the management of peripheral arterial disease PAOD, however, most studies have been uncontrolled or small and are now regarded with some cynicism [23] thus the role of pharmacotherapy in CLI is not yet clearly defined. Nevertheless, some of the pathophysiological considerations of CLI suggest a theoretical role for such medicines and this article reviews these and summarises the clinical studies in severe limb ischaemia. Unfortunately, few reported studies deal with patients who suffer from CLI as defined by the European Working Group [37]. Extrapolation from less selected groups of patients is therefore unavoidable. Nevertheless, pharmacotherapeutic approaches can be broadly divided into primary medical management, adjunctive pharmacotherapy after grafting or angioplasty, and the management of risk factors/disease progression. These will be evaluated in turn.

Blood Constituents and Critical Limb Ischaemia

The role of platelets in the formation of arterial thromboses has been well described [43]. Platelets may be activated either as a primary event or whilst passing over atherosclerotic plaques or through post-stenotic vortices in the proximal arteries. Thus the already prejudiced limb can be perfused with a high proportion of activated cells. Activated platelets release vasoconstrictive substances such as thromboxane A_2 (TXA_2) and serotonin, physical aggregates are formed which may aggravate the disease further by obstructing the microvasculature. Circulating platelet aggregates have been detected in CLI [43] as have increased levels of the stable metabolite of TXA_2, TXB_2 [18]. Other platelet release products have also been detected in increased amounts in CLI and parallel the well documented increased rate of platelet aggregation [43].

The haemorheology of other blood cells has also been studied. The diameter of the red blood cell (RBC) is approximately 5 microns and this is greater than that of some of the capillaries in the microcirculation. Thus blood flow may be critically dependent on RBC deformability. In the ischaemic limb, RBC aggregation is further increased under the reduced temperature, low shear/low flow, conditions [59]. Increased RBC number is, furthermore, inversely correlated with arterial graft survival [18]. These findings led to the suggestion that decreased whole blood filtrability in PAOD was secondary to increased RBC rigidity. However, newer tests involving removal of white blood cell (WBC) contamination combined with measures of WBC deformability, suggest that the predominant influence in decreased whole blood filtration in CLI is the increased rigidity of the activated WBC [24]. Indeed, the WBC count is a predictor of future amputation rate in CLI [5].

Polymorphonuclear leukocytes (PMNs) are about 2000 times less deformable than erythrocytes [12]. When they become activated they project pseudopods and their cytoplasmic stiffness increases further. Adhesion to the blood vessel wall can occlude the vessel and adhesion to other cells, including other WBCs, can lead to the formation of microaggregates. Once the WBC has become fixed in the microcirculation it can delivery a variety of further insults to the vessel lining including the release of

96

toxic oxygen metabolites, some of which are free radicals (FRs). Patients with PAOD have decreased radical scavengers in their blood and increased products of FR activity [12] which are further augmented by exercise [48], or immediately after ischaemia reperfusion such as occurs during the process of angioplasty [57].

The blood plasma is also important in contributing to blood flow in critical limb ischaemia. Blood factors that are important in thrombus formation in the arteries must, of course, include the blood clotting factors and there is some suggestion that young vasculopaths may have an unrecognised thrombophilia in the form of congenital deficiencies of protein C and protein S. Although these factors are more usually associated with venous thromboembolism they may be relevant in arterial thrombosis [72]. Protein C is a vitamin K-dependent inhibitor of coagulation which, in activated form, acts as a potent anticoagulant, by inhibiting the activated clotting factors V and VIII. Protein S is another vitamin K-dependent factor and it is a co-factor for protein C, augmenting its inhibitory activity.

Several epidemiological studies have confirmed that fibrinogen, another blood clotting factor, is an important independent predictor of cardiovascular events [87]. Fibrinogen may promote such cardiovascular disease through several potential mechanisms including increased fibrin formation, platelet aggregation, infiltration of the vessel wall and plasma viscosity. Patients with PAOD have elevated plasma fibrinogen levels and these may be of prognostic value [32]. There is a further increase in the fibrinogen level in CLI [59] which may influence the longer term patency of vein grafts [87]. The deposition of fibrin, however, is not only dependent upon fibrinogen level but is modified by the activation and inhibition of fibrinolysis. Two important participators in the lysis of fibrin are produced by the endothelium.

The Endothelium and Critical Limb Ischaemia

The endothelium is a functioning organ releasing important chemicals. It has an important role in preventing inappropriate thombosis whilst maintaining haemostasis. Plasma fibrinolysis is largely controlled by the endothelium through its ability to produce tissue plasminogen activator (tPA) and plasminogen activator inhibitor (PAI). The activation of plasminogen to plasmin is promoted by tPA. Fibrin is then lysed by plasmin. PAOD patients have impaired fibrinolysis which may favour atherogenesis, arterial thrombosis and microemboli formation [27].

Prostacyclin (PGI_2) is another endothelial product. Work investigating endothelial production of PGI_2 in PAOD was hindered initially by the difficulty in measuring the stable metabolite 6-keto $PGF_1\alpha$. Animal studies reported a bi-phasic response of the endothelium during the development of experimental atherosclerosis with an initial increase during the early stages as the endothelium mounted a protective response, and a late decrease in production reflecting endothelial cell dysfunction [4]. This work probably explains the clinical findings of increased prostacyclin production in PAOD [39] but decreased production of PGI_2 from atheromatous plaque in CLI [27].

Other endothelial products may be altered in CLI. PAOD patients have increased plasma levels of Factor VIII von Willebrand Factor Antigen (VWF) [10] which not only marks vascular damage but can propagate the disease by participation in the coagulation cascade and by promoting platelet aggregation. Endothelium-derived relaxing factor (EDRF, NO) is another endothelium-derived vasodilator. It is also difficult to measure, as are endothelial vasoconstrictors such as endothelin. Results from studies in CLI of these substances are awaited.

Pharmacotherapy for critical limb ischaemia

Theoretical considerations

The majority of hemorheological abnormalities detected in CLI can be found to a lesser extent in patients with intermittent claudication or in subjects with risk factors for PAOD [20, 52]. Thus the majority of these are likely to be a consequence of the vessel damage rather than the direct cause. The exception to this is possibly the WBC, whose count is a prospective marker for vascular disease with the same degree of certainty as a single cholesterol measure or test of blood pressure [41]. Nevertheless, impaired endothelial cell function, activated WBCs or platelets±hard red cells will contribute to impaired flow in the microcirculation in CLI and their correction by pharmacotherapy could produce clinical improvement.

Medical management alone, as a treatment for critical limb ischaemia

Vasodilator anti-platelet prostaglandins

Anti-platelet vasodilator therapies might be expected to be useful in a disease characterised by abnormal vasomotor activity and platelet aggregation [89]. An initial concern that such potent vasodilators might produce a "steal" effect through vasodilation in vascular beds elsewhere, proved unfounded in PAOD. Additionally some of the prostaglandins have been shown to increase fibrinolysis [83], probably in a passive fashion as a result of intense vasodilatation. An abnormal fibrinolytic response to venous occlusion in PAOD has been normalised by the prostacyclin analogue iloprost [15]. Some early reports suggested that the prostaglandins may increase red cell deformability [34], others have found no effect or even decreased filterability [7]. This variation may reflect either differences in the prostaglandins used or the effects of the prostaglandins on platelets and leukocytes which may have contaminated the test erythrocyte suspensions. This latter suggestion is thought to be the most likely as PGI_2 has profound antiplatelet effects and also modifies WBC behaviour [9].

Prostacyclin

The first published work supporting the use of native PGI_2 as a treatment for CLI was encouraging although the study was uncontrolled [77]. Later double-blind placebo-controlled studies did, however, support the results [8, 55]. The response produced, however, was at best seen only short-term in carefully selected patients, and in other studies PGI_2 appeared only equipotent with naftidrofuryl [54]. Furthermore, PGI_2 requires careful storage, handling and preparation. It is unstable and of short duration of action. It must be freshly prepared and given by continuous intravenous (IV) infusion. Other problems, associated with the IV administration of any drug can also occur, for example, infection at the site of the cannula insertion. This

98

Table 1. Prostaglandin doses used in critical limb ischaemia

	Maximum dose	Route	Daily infusion length	Treatment period
Prostacyclin	7.5 ng/kg/min	IV	8 hours	21 infusions over 28 days
Iloprost	2 ng/kg/min	IV	6 hours	21 infusions over 28 days
Prostaglandin E_1	10–20 ng/kg/min or 60 µg/day	IV	8 hours	21 daily infusions
Lipo-PGE$_1$	10 µg	IV	5 minutes	20 injections over 28 days

is in addition to the local side effects occurring if there is leakage of the prostaglandin from the cannula into the tissue. The PGs narrow therapeutic window also means that patients have to be carefully monitored with slow incremental increases in dosage to a maximum tolerated dose which can vary from patient to patient (Table 1). Although serious side-effects are uncommon using the correct dosage regime, most patients will experience facial flushing and headache. A few will require a decrease in drug dosage usually because of nausea, some may vomit and occasionally hypotension occurs. These problems would be tolerable if the treatment were curative. Unfortunately, in our experience, repetition of the regime is required at varying intervals with all the above attendant problems.

Iloprost

One of the newer prostacyclin analogues, iloprost, addresses one of these problems, it is a carbacyclin derivative of prostacyclin and is chemically stable, it appears equipotent to PGI_2 in its antiplatelet effects. In most studies, like PGI_2, it also has anti-WBC activity [9]. Its chemical stability means it retains more than 95% of its antiplatelet activity after 7 days at room temperature and though still currently being given IV, its stability makes its use much more convenient. Early placebo controlled studies of iloprost treatment in CLI suggested a clinical potency equal to that of PGI_2 [49, 59]. The individually tolerated doses of iloprost were assessed in the first three days of treatment by stepwise titration of the dose which was then held constant throughout the study time period. The doses investigated were never above 2 ng/kg/min and the infusions lasted for 6 h/day for a full length of 14–28 days.

Six major randomised double blind controlled studies using iloprost in CLI have so far been undertaken [21, 30, 38, 40, 47, 57] (Table 1). In the first German multicenter study [30], 101 patients were given iloprost for 28 days, 17% of the placebo group had partial or complete healing of their ulcers versus 61.5% in the iloprost group ($p < 0.05$). The treatment effect persisted in both groups for at least 1 year (24% versus 55%). Partial healing was defined as "partial but distinctly visible healing of the largest ulcer" at the end of the 4 weeks of therapy. The second placebo controlled German study [21] enrolled 109 diabetic patients. At the end of 28 days, 23.5% of the placebo group had responded versus 62% of the iloprost group.

The Scandinavian/Polish study [57] enrolled 103 patients with CLI into their 6-month study. The patients received 2 weeks of iloprost or placebo treatment. The response rate in the placebo group was 25% versus 41.3% in the iloprost treated group (p = 0.086). For this study the response definition was healing of at least one-third of the ulcer area after 6 months and the authors concluded that the 2-week infusion period was too short.

The French multicenter study [47] investigated 128 patients of whom 74 were diabetic. Iloprost was given for 6 h for 21 days by continuous IV infusion. Rest pain had disappeared at day 28 in 19% of placebo treated patients compared to 50% of patients in the iloprost group (p < 0.05). Analgesic consumption was significantly lower in the iloprost group at day 60.

In the UK, a study of 151 patients [40] investigated 64 Fontaine stage III patients who were treated for 14 days and 87 Fontaine stage IV (CLI) patients for 28 days. Overall results showed clinical efficacy in 29% of the placebo group compared to 45% of patients treated with iloprost (p < 0.05). The authors concluded that duration of treatment was important as those patients treated for 28 days appeared to improve significantly more than those treated for 14 days.

Finally, an aspirin controlled study of iloprost in thromboangitis obliterans (Buerger's disease) has also been reported [38]. 133 patients were treated for 28 days and a response was seen in 17% of the patients on aspirin compared to 85% of the patients receiving iloprost. The definition of response was complete relief of ischaemic pain or ulcer healing of over 50% of the ulcer area.

These studies have been criticised for the "softness" of their end-points, i.e. relief of rest pain and ulcer healing. It should be remembered, however, that the hard end-points such as amputation rate and mortality would need very large patient numbers. It is of interest that a meta-analysis of the five CLI studies that evaluated atherosclerotic CLI has shown an increase in ulcer healing (p < 0.04) and a reduction in amputation rate by about half at 3 – 6 months in CLI patients treated with iloprost (p < 0.05) [28]. Where mortality data was available the combination of two major end-points (amputation and death rate) from these trials strengthened the suggestion of benefit from iloprost. Indeed the meta-analysis showed that iloprost almost halved the incidence of these combined end-points.

Prostaglandin E_1

As with prostacyclin, intravenous administration of PGE_1 was initially studied over a relatively short period of 3 days. These studies did not result in a significant benefit for the patient [36, 53, 73, 79]. In contrast, however, the use of intermittent PGE_1 therapy over a longer period of 3/4 weeks resulted in the same type of benefits as have been seen with iloprost [29, 82] (Table 1). The study by Diehm et al. [29] was double-blinded placebo controlled whilst that by Trubestein et al. [82] was controlled by pentoxifylline. Both studies also resulted in reduced analgesic consumption and pain relief.

As an endogenous substance, PGE_1 is rapidly metabolised during first passage through the lungs. Sixty to ninety percent of the given dose of PGE_1 is metabolised to 15-keto-PGE_1, 15-keto 13, 14-dyhydro-PGE_1 and 13, 14-dyhydro-PGE_1 (PGE_0). It was initially thought, therefore, that it was likely to be less potent than prostacyclin which is not so metabolised. However, unlike the 15-keto-metabolites which are less active, the pharmacodynamic spectrum of PGE_0 closely resembles that of PGE_1 and might contribute to the therapeutic efficacy outlined above. One of the major drawbacks, however, in the use of PGE_1 is a necessity to infuse the substance via a central line because of the development of severe thrombophlebitis in peripheral veins. This handling difficulty, combined with the larger doses that must be given due to its high elimination rate after the first pass through the lung, increases the incidence of adverse effects. Based upon experience with liposomes as drug carriers, the Green Cross Corporation, Osaka, Japan, developed lipo-PGE_1. The lipid part of the formulation is similar to the lipid infusions which have been used for over 20 year for parenteral nutrition. Because of lipo-encapsulation, the PGE_1 is protected from the first pass effect and can be used in much lower doses compared to native PGE_1 [81]. The lipid particles are metabolised in a similar way to chylomicrons and because of their affinity for the vessel wall, they carry PGE_1 to the target tissue in PAOD. Lipo-PGE_1 has been compared favourably with PGE_1 in small pilot studies in PAOD [66, 88] being administered as a once daily bolus IV injection thus allowing the patients to be treated as out-patients. Future results from large multicentre studies are awaited on this compound.

Other antiplatelet agents

The use of antiplatelet agents such as aspirin, dipyridamole and ticlopidine have proven disappointing in the management of critical limb ischaemia as primary pharmacotherapy. The exception to this is the syndrome of recurrent attacks of pain and cyanosis in the toes, and sometimes fingers, which has been associated with thrombocytosis and evidence of increased platelet activity. The distal pulses are normal and it is thought that microvascular ischaemia may arise from platelet aggregation, a hypothesis supported by the beneficial clinical response to aspirin [86]. Thus whilst there is no role for such agents as primary pharmacotherapy for CLI this should not detract from their potential prophylactic role as regards coronary and cerebral events and disease progression. Furthermore, there is probably a role for such agents as adjunctive therapy to distal grafting and angioplasty (See later).

Dextran

Intravenous infusion of dextran has been advocated in the treatment of rest pain or pre-gangrene. Contrary to popular belief, dextrans have no specific effect on blood viscosity, in fact, the high molecular weight dextran molecules increase the viscosity of plasma. This effect is counter-balanced by a fall in haematocrit and hence in whole blood viscosity due to the diluting effect of the infused fluid and also to a further increase in plasma volume as the hyperosmolar a extran draws in further fluid from the extravascular space. Thus dextran reduces blood viscosity by hemodilution [31]. Peripheral blood flow does appear to increase acutely following dextran infusion. This is probably a consequence of hypervolaemia rather than a reduction in blood viscosity and nutritional blood flow is not increased [46]. Clinical benefit from dextran infusion has yet to be assessed in major controlled trials and this should be remembered when considering its use. It can produce serious adverse effects such as pulmonary oedema in patients with impaired cardiac reserve. Other adverse effects include anaphylaxis, bleeding, and renal failure.

Hemodilution with a replacement fluid less likely to cause to above effects has been assessed in PAOD though the majority of work has been undertaken in those with Fontaine Stage II and III disease [56]. Studies suggesting improvement in ischaemic skin ulceration and in patients undergoing limited amputation suggest that a large controlled study could be worthwhile in this situation [3]. A direct comparison with one of the prostaglandins should be incorporated into the study design. A full review of this area however is outwith the remit of this article.

Fibrinogen and fibrinolysis

As discussed previously fibrinogen reduction allows a decrease in plasma viscosity and red cell aggregation. These two effects produce a reduction in whole blood viscosity particularly at the low shear rates which favour red cell aggregation. Disappointingly controlled studies of initially promising defibrinating agents derived from snake-venom, e.g. ancrod, have been disappointing [58].

Of more interest, however, is the use of thrombolytic agents in acute critical limb ischaemia. Surgical removal of a pheripheral arterial thrombus using a Fogarty catheter is usually considered the first and fastest therapeutic approach. However, the short-term and long-term success rates of thrombectomy are low in an atherosclerotic artery and this technique is less often successful when treatment is delayed for 24 hours, or when the thrombus is distal to the popliteal artery [1]. Vascular reconstruction or local endarterectomy may then be tried. More recently, however, the use of local thrombolysis has been employed. Streptokinase, urokinase, tissue type plasminogen activator and anistreplase (anisoylated plasminogen-streptokinase activator) are commercially availabe. Local treatment with low-dose streptokinase or urokinase infused into the blood clot is successful in about $50-80\%$ of patients [13, 51] and recanalization is sustained for up to one year in approximately 50% [56]. Plasminogen activator treatment produces a similar profile of results, however, although the dosages used in thrombolytic therapy are low (streptokinase 5000 IU/h, urokinase 60000 IU/h or tPA 0.5 to 1 mg/h), the risk of minor bleeding is $15-20\%$ and of major haemorrhage 10% [42]. Ricotta et al. [71] collected the results of 623 patients who had been treated outside clinical trials. The success rate, defined as reperfusion resulting in a viable limb, was 50% but there were serious complications in 20% including a mortality rate of 2.3%, stroke (1.4%) and leg amputation (15%). These findings may reflect everyday experience more accurately than trials in specialized vascular centres. Our own experience with approximately 100 patients requiring thrombolysis is that success can be achieved in approximately 50% of cases. We have combined this with 4 to 6 hourly monitoring of blood coagulation. The infusion is stopped temporarily if the fibrinogen level falls significantly, and the dose of the lytic agent increased if the fibrinogen is maintained and the fibrin degradation product levels fail to increase. In this way we believe that we are achieving optimum lyses with a good safety profile (3% bleeding incidence, 0% mortality). These safety measures are combined in our centre with absolute contra-indications which include factors that could contribute to intra-cranial bleeding such as a recent history of stroke or transient ischaemic attack, other intra-cranial lesions or uncontrolled hypertension. The guidelines for patient selection are broadly the same as those for myocardial infarction and must be strictly adhered to. Little information is available regarding the advisability or otherwise of full anticoagulation following thrombolysis. In our experience the majority of patients require angioplasty for a stenotic lesion underlying the thrombus and it is our routine practice to carry this out, under full heparinization, and to subsequently warfarinize the patients for a variable period depending on the residual run-off.

Thrombolytic therapy is a potentially promising treatment for acute critical limb ischaemia if there is a suitably recent and sited thrombus. Clinical experience suggests a role for such treatment in selected patients, however, there is the need for further well designed clinical studies. It is important that thrombolytic treatment be compared to surgical intervention. Disappointingly a study assessing this using tPA as the lytic agent and surgery as the comparator, has recently been stopped due to poor enrolment numbers. This is not surprising as it is our experience that those patients referred for thrombolysis are those in which surgery appears to be the greater risk. As the study was a blind randomization to surgery or thrombolysis, such patients would not be suitable for enrolment. At the present time it is considered useful in carefully selected patients with recent onset of thrombus formation or graft thrombosis.

Anticoagulants

Despite the fact that some rare cases of protein C and S deficiency may present with arterial thrombus there is, in general, no benefit from primary treatment of CLI with warfarin. In the acute limb, particularly if the occlusion is embolic in nature, immediate full heparinization can induce clinical benefit. In general, however, primary heparin treatment of chronic critical limb ischaemia is ineffective.

Vasodilators

Oral vasodilators are of no proven value in critical limb ischaemia. In severe ischaemia vasodilation may already be maximal due to hypoxia. Drug induced vasodilation in other tissues may then divert blood away from areas of critical ischaemia, the so-called "steal" effect. One of the more commonly used vasodilators is naftidrofuryl and whilst it is not the place of this review to document its effects in intermittent claudication, it is available as an intravenously administered preparation and is used in CLI. In addition to its vasodilatory effects it is thought to enhance metabolism in ischaemia tissue [74] and may have rheological effects. Some small double blind controlled studies of naftidrofuryl versus placebo for ischaemic rest pain have suggested some benefit from this compound [17, 78]. Although the latter study did not alter the outcome in patients with rest pain and merely afforded symptomatic relief for a period of time, this symptomatic improvement by the use of naftidrofuryl was also seen in a later study [52], comparing symptom relief in CLI using bed rest and heating, versus bed rest heating and intravenous naftidrofuryl. It is of interest that a comparative study with PGI_2 suggests that naftidrofuryl is equipotent to prostacyclin [54]. At the present time it is difficult to critically assess the data relating to the use of intravenous naftidrofuryl in CLI. It is important that well designed studies similar to those carried out with iloprost are assessed in this area and in view of the discrepancies in the cost between such a compound and the prostaglandins, we would suggest that the comparator should be a prostaglandin.

Adjunctive pharmacotherapy in critical limb ischaemia

Graft Patency

Many vascular surgeons prescribe antiplatelet drugs for a prolonged period of time post-operatively in the hope of improving their graft patency rates. Data to substantiate this practice is however sparce. Recommendations are usually based on conclusions of Consensus Documents [37] or on meta-analysis of pooled data. For example, one working group suggested the administration of antiplatelet therapy (aspirin 325 mg plus dipyridamole 225 mgs) to patients having prosthetic or saphenous vein femoropopliteal bypass operations [25, 44]. This advise however was based on an evaluation of four published randomised trials but the study population in these trials include a mixture of vein grafts and prosthetic grafts. Three of the studies where antiplatelet therapy was started before surgery suggested benefit from such antiplatelet therapy although one of them suggested that the effect was limited to prosthetic grafts and confined to the first post-operative month. The fourth study found no difference between active and placebo but treatment was started after surgery only. In contrast the Second Cycle report of the Antiplatelet Trialists' Collaboration meta-analysed 12 randomised trials including over 2000 patients with peripheral vascular grafts [2]. Antiplatelet drugs reduced the incidence of graft occlusion at the end of the variable follow-up period by a factor of one-third (from 25 to 16%). The latest study to evaluate antiplatelet drugs in femoropopliteal vein bypasses suggested no benefit [50] and it would appear that at present the impression is that antiplatelet therapy is only clearly effective for synthetic grafts. To a certain extent this argument is academic as antiplatelet therapy should probably be instituted in these patients in an effort to modify the risk of cardio- and cerebrovascular events (See later).

A major determinant of graft blood flow is the peripheral resistance in the run off-bed. In the presence of an adequate inflow this appears to have a strong predictive value for graft failure. The microcirculation makes a major contribution to vascular outflow resistance in the ischaemic leg and this can be influenced by a number of factors most of which are worsened by reperfusion injury of the leg which occurs on completion of arterial reconstruction. The initial adverse effects of restoration of blood flow in the microcirculation explains the delay in achieving maximum flow and may contribute to early graft failure. It would therefore seem advantageous to decrease microvascular resistance at the time of arterial reconstruction and so achieve maximum early graft bed flow. Shearman et al. [74] have investigated 3000 ng of iloprost given as a single local infusion over 2 min via an unligated side branch in the proximal end of the vein graft. The study was double blind and placebo controlled and blood flow volume was measured with an electromagnetic flow probe. Duplex ultrasound scanning for 7 days after surgery provided the follow-up. A marked increase in graft blood flow was noted in patients receiving iloprost was noted and this was still apparent at 7 days. The relative risk of graft occlusion for the iloprost group was significantly less during the first month than for placebo. Although during the following year iloprost grafts tended to fair better, they did not do so in a statistically significant fashion and the longer term effects of this treatment need further evaluation.

Angioplasty

In the last decade percutaneous transluminal angioplasty (PTA) has become widely accepted as a treatment for CLI particularly in the elderly and medically unfit patient with extensive disease. The longer term benefits of PTA have, however, been limited by restenosis of the dilated segment and restenosis rates follwoing PTA in the femoropopliteal segments of the peripheral vessels range from 20−84% in different reported series [26, 53]. Platelet activation and adherence to de-endothelialised surfaces is thought to contribute to this restenosis particularly in the early stages. However, various antiplatelet agents have failed to prevent the appearance of a later restenotic lesion [50]. It has been suggested that the mechanism of restenosis is more consistent with the response to injury hypothesis whereby platelet deposition causes release of growth factors. Thus antiplatelet agents will decrease the incidence of acute thrombosis following PTA but may not have any effect on the longer term restenosis rate. In support of this, clinical evidence of the efficacy and need for antiplatelet agents is poorly documented. The effects of aspirin are better documented in coronary angioplasty but the question remains as to whether data from coronary procedures can be extrapolated to the peripheral circulation. Properly controlled trials addressing the need for long-term antiplatelet therapy are rare. Four trials were recently reviewed [85], the general impression was that antiplatelet drugs had little influence on the late recurrence of stenosis or occlusion. Despite this, and similar to the argument relating to vascular grafting, there is logical and sound argument supporting the use of antiplatelet drugs in patients with CLI as prophylaxis against secondary vascular events and this renders the above argument academic.

We, ourselves have been evaluating omega 6 and omega 3 essential fatty acids as therapy to prevent restenosis. These essential fatty acids have potent antiplatelet effects and, in addition, can modify the body's inflammatory response to injury and may thus have an effect on the later occlusion rate resultant from smooth muscle cell proliferation and neo-intimal proliferation [79]. A 1-year treatment regime produced a restenosis rate of 17% in the treated group compared to 48% in the placebo group [6]. A multicentre double blind study is currently underway to evaluate this treatment.

Risk factor management and/or disease progression in CLI

In general patients with PAOD have a reduced life expectancy because of the associated high risk of coronary artery and cerebrovascular disease. Those patients with intermittent claudication have, on average, a 5% yearly mortality which is 2−3 times higher than expected. In patients with CLI the prognosis is even worse with a 10−20% annual mortality [80]. In addition, there is a considerable risk of non fatal coronary and cerebrovascular events [33].

Support for the beneficial effect of antiplatelet drugs comes from a meta-analysis of 28 smaler trials involving patients with PAOD. A total of 3864 patients were enrolled in the study and 444 vascular events occurred. Antiplatelet agents reduced the risk of experiencing a vascular event (both fatal an non fatal) by 25±10% [2]. Whether patients with a high risk profile, such as those with CLI, experience a greater or lesser benefit from antiplatelet therapy is however at present unknown. Aspirin has been best studied but in recent years ticlopidine has been studied as a new agent.

Table 2. Risk factors for the development and progression of blood flow disturbances

Smoking
Diabetis mellitus
Hypertension
Hyperlipidaemia
Obesity
Lack of physical exercise

A meta-analysis of four trials indicated that this drug reduced the instance of fatal and non fatal vascular events from 9 to 3% in a total of 611 patients observed for between 6–12 months [16] and another study has shown that ticlopidine reduced the mortality rate by 29% and cardiac mortality by 43% [51]. Thus it is fairly certain that antiplatelet therapy confers some protection against secondary vascular events as measured by cardiac mortality and non fatal cardiac events. What is less clear is whether antiplatelet agents themselves inhibit progression of the peripheral arterial disease itself.

A number of studies have suggested that aspirin ± dipyridamole, or ticlopidine are effective in retarding the progression of atherosclerosis and preventing thrombotic complications in the legs. Due to inconsistencies in patients' selection, however, and absence of measurable clinical end-points, no clear consensus has emerged from these studies [84]. The American work showing the delayed development of PAOD in subjects taking aspirin as a cardio-protective agent is of interest therefore, and further work is required in this area.

Some of the risk factors that are well established for cardiovascular disease may also play a role in peripheral arterial disease (Table 2) and whilst some of these, such as exercise and smoking cessation, are not addressed pharmacologically, others may be relevant in a review such as this. This includes the introduction of appropriate lipid-lowering agents and the diagnosis and management of diabetes. Elevated plasma levels of cholesterol and triglycerides are associated with vascular disease in general and it is generally agreed that lipid-lowering agents are effective in reducing cardiac mortality. With the advent of the newer, more powerful agents, progression of the disease in the coronary vessels appears to have been halted and possibly even decreased [22]. Hyperlipidaemia should be managed appropriately in patients with PAOD as these elevated lipids certainly play a role in coronary artery disease and it is likely that they also contribute to disease in the extremity. Policy guidelines for the selection of patients requiring therapy have been issued by the European Atherosclerosis Society [70] and as these have been made widely available throughout Europe we do not propose to document them in this review. Detection and management of diabetes is also important and it is well recognised that a poorly controlled diabetic is at a much greater risk for development of peripheral arterial disease. Potent hypoglycaemic agents are available and, as with lipid-lowering therapy, should be combined with an appropriate diet.

Another risk factor which is associated with PAOD is hypertension with both elevated levels of systolic blood pressure being associated with its development. Treatment of hypertension has been shown to reduce the incidence of stroke, heart failure and renal failure and it is, therefore, justified to introduce antihypertensive therapy in patients with critical limb ischaemia in an effort to prevent secondary vascular

Table 3. Factors affecting nutritional flow

Perfusion = $\dfrac{\text{Flow conditions}}{\text{Flow properties}}$		perfusion pressure ↑ cardiac output ↑ whole blood viscosity ↓ platelet aggregation ↓ white cell activity ↓

events elsewhere. It should be noted, however, that an elevated blood pressure in the early phase of CLI may be contributing to perfusion of the affected limb. Therefore a difficult balance has to be maintained to ensure adequate limb perfusion but yet still limit the risk of stroke. The Consensus Document on CLI [37] recommends that antihypertensive treatment should not be instituted in the early stage in patients whose systolic blood pressure in the standing or sitting position is lower than 180 mmHg and diastolic blood pressure lower than 100 mmHg. It should be remembered that conventional beta blockers may have a deleterious effect on peripheral blood flow, although newer vasodilatory beta blockers are now available. In general however, if treatment of hypertension is necessary calcium antagonists, angiotensin converting enzyme (ACE) inhibitors or other vasodilating substances should be used.

A high proportion of patients with CLI have other co-existent diseases especially cardiovascular and respiratory disorders. These latter occur due to the higher proportion of smokers in this patient population. Pharmacotherapy for co-existent cardiac disease such as heart failure and arrhythmia will improve pump function and may improve perfusion pressure in the critically ischaemic limb [76] (Table 3). A chest infection may lower blood oxygenation and should be aggressively treated. Local infection at the site of the limb ischaemia should also be actively treated and oedema should be noted and, where necessary, treated with a mild diuretic.

Conclusion

Vascular reconstructive surgery is the therapeutic choice in patients with limb-threatening ischaemia. Vascular surgery should be considered even in the elderly patient with CLI. This is supported by the Consensus Document [3] which recommends that a reconstructive procedure should be attempted "so long as there is a reasonable chance of saving a useful limb in a patient who has evidence of sufficient run-off and who is fit for surgery". Graft surveillance to detect the 20−30% of stenosis occurring within one year of surgery has improved patient outcome to the degree that surgery is the "gold standard" treatment for CLI [19]. Nevertheless, for those patients not suitable for surgery some form of pharmacotherapy may be useful, in particular, the vasodilatory antiplatelet prostaglandins. Furthermore, in those patients in whom surgery is undertaken, medical managements as an adjunct to the surgery or endovascular procedure may also be useful. Finally, although critical limb ischaemia has a high morbidity, the mortality is usually from cardiac or cerebral events and secondary prevention of these events by modification or risk factors and judicious use of antiplatelet therapy should be encouraged in all patients with critical limb ischaemia.

Acknowledgements

Dr. J. J. F. Belch is supported by the Sir John Fisher Foundation.

References

1. Abbott WM, McCabe C, Maloney RD, Wirthlin LS (1984) Embolism of the popliteal artery. Surg Gynecol Obstet 159:533−536
2. Antiplatelet Trialists' Collaboration (1988) Secondary prevention of vascular disease by prolonged antiplatelet treatment. Br Med J 296:320−331
3. Bailey MJ, Yates CJP, Johnston CLW, Somerville PG, Dormandy JA (1979) Pre-operative haemoglobin as predictor of outcome of diabetic amputations. Lancet ii:168−170
4. Beetens JR, Coene M-C, Verheyen A, Zonnekeyn L, Herman AG (1986) Biphasic response of intimal prostacyclin production during the development of experimental atherosclerosis. Prostaglandins 32(3):319−334
5. Belch JJF, Diehm C, Söhngen W, Frings M: The leucocyte count as a prognostic factor in critical limb ischaemia (submitted for publication)
6. Belch JJF, Schaw JW, Lau CS, McConachie NS, Mackay IR, Stewart JCM (in press) Restenosis following percutaneous transluminal balloon angioplasty for peripheral arterial disease: A double-blind controlled trial of omega 6/omega 3 essential fatty acids
7. Belch JJF, Lowe GDO, Drummond MM, Forbes CD, Prentice CRM (1981) Prostacyclin reduces red cell deformability. Thromb Haemostas 45:189
8. Belch JJF, McArdle B, Pollock JG, Forbes CD, McKay A, Leiberman P, Lower GDO, Prentice CRM (1983) Epoprostenol (prostacyclin) and severe arterial disease: double-blind trial. Lancet; February 12:315−317
9. Belch JJF, Saniabadi A, Forbes CD (1986) The effect of ZK36374 (Iloprost) on white cell behaviour. In: Prostacyclin and its Stable Analogue Iloprost. Schror K, Gryglewski RJ (eds) Springer Verlag: Berlin 97:102
10. Belch JJF, Zoma A, Richards I, Forbes CD, Sturrock RD (1987) Vascular damage and factor VIII related antigen in the rheumatic disease. Rheumatol Int 7:107−111
11. Belch JJF, Ansell D, Madhok R, O'Dowd A, Sturrock RD (1988) Effects of altering dietary essential fatty acids on requirements for non-steroidal drugs in patients with rheumatoid arthritis. Ann Rheum Dis 47:96−99
12. Belch JJF, Chopra M, Hutchison S, Lorimer R, Sturrock RD, Forbes CD, Smith WE (1989) Free radical pathology ain chronic arterial disease. Free Rad Biol Med 6:375−378
13. Belch JJF, Mackay I, Hillis S (1993) Thrombolytic therapy in arterial disease: II. thrombolysis and peripheral arterial occlusion. Vascular Medicine Review 4(2):111−115
14. Bell P, London N (1992) Surgical treatment of critical ischaemia. Crit Ischaem 2(1):15−23
15. Bertele V, Mussoni L, Del Rosso G (1988) Defective fibrinolytic response in atherosclerotic patients. Effect of iloprost and its possible mechanism of action. Thromb Haemostas 60:141−144
16. Boissel JP, Peyrieux JC, Destors JM (1989) Is it possible to reduce the risk of cardiovascular events in subjects suffering from intermittent claudication of the lower limbs? Thrombosis and Haemostatis 62:681−685
17. Boobis LH, Bell PRF (1982) Can drugs help patients with lower limb ischaemia. Brit J Surg 69:17−23
18. Bouhoutsos J, Morris T, Chavatzas D, Martin P (1974) The influence of haemoglobin and platelet levels on the results of arterial surgery. Br J Surg 61:984−986
19. Brennan JA, Thrush A, Evans DH, Bell PRF (1991) Perioperative monitoring of blood flow in femoro infragenicular vein grafts with Doppler ultrasonography: A preliminary report. J Vasc Surg 13(4):468−475
20. Bridges AB, Hill A, Belch JJF (1993) Cigarette smoking increases white blood cell aggregation in whole blood. J R Soc Med 86:139−140
21. Broch FE, Abri O, Baitsch G, Bechara G, Beck K (1990) Iloprost in der Behandlung ischamischer Gewelsslasionen bei Diabetikern. Schweizerische Med Wochenschrift 120: 1477−1482

22. Brown G, Albers JJ, Fisher LD, Schaefer SM, Lin J-T, Kaplan C, Zaho X-Q, Bisson BD, Fitz-patrick VF, Doge HT (1990) Regression of coronary artery disease as a rsult of intensive lipid-lowering therapy in men with high levels of apolipoprotein B. N Engl J Med 323 (November 8):1289–1298

23. Cameron HA, Waller PC, Ramsay LE (1988) Drug treatment of intermittent claudication: A critical analysis of the methods and findings of published clinical trials, 1965–1985. Br J Clin Pharmac 26:569–576

24. Ciuffetti G, Mercuri M, Mannarino E, Robinson MK, Lennie SE, Lowe G (1989) Peripheral vascular disease. Rheologic variables during controlled ischemia. Circulation 80(2):348–352

25. Clagett GP, Genton E, Salzman EW (1989) Antithrombotic therapy in peripheral vascular disease. Chest 95:128S–139S

26. Cumberland DC (1983) Percutaneous transluminal angioplasty: a review. Clin Radiol 34:25–38

27. D'Angelo Y, Villa S, Mysllvvlec M, Donati MB, de Gaetano G (1978) Defective fibrinolytic and prostacyclin-like activity in human atheromatous plaques. Thromb Haemostas 39:535–536

28. de Gaetano G, Cerletti C, Bertele' V (1992) The use of prostanoids in critical limb ischaemia. Crit Ischaem 2(2):5–12

29. Diehm C, Hübsch-Müller C, Stammler F (1988) Intravenöse Prostaglandin E_1-Therapie bei Patienten mit peripherer arterieller Verschlußkrankheit (AVK) im Stadium III – eine doppelblinde, plazebokontrollierte Studie. In: Heidrich H, Bohme H, Rogatti W (eds) Prostaglandin E_1-Wirkung and therapeutische Wirksamkeit. Heidelberg: Springer, 133–143

30. Diehm C, Abri O, Baitsch G, Bechara G, Beck K, Breddin HK, Brock FE, Clevert HD, Corovic D, Marshall M, Rahmel B, Scheffler P, Schmidt W, Oberender HA (1989) Iloprost, ein stabiles Prostacyclinderivat, bei arterieller Verschlußkrankheit im Stadium IV. Dtsch Med Wschr 114:783–788

31. Dormandy JA (1971) Influence of blood viscosity on blood flow an the effect of low molecular weight dextran. British Medical Journal 4:716–719

32. Dormandy JA, Hoare E, Colley J, Arrowsmith DE, Dormandy TL (1973) Clinical, haemodynamic, rheological, and biochemical findings in 126 patients with intermittent claudication. Brit Med J, December 576–581

33. Dormandy J, Mahr M, Ascady G (1989) Fate of the patient with chronic leg ischaemia. A review article. J Cardiovasc Surg 30:55–57

34. Dowd PM, Kovacs IB, Bland CJH, Kirby JDT (1981) Effect of prostaglandins I_2 and E_1 on red cell deformability in patients with Raynaud's phenomenon and systemic sclerosis. Brit Med J 283:350

35. Eikelboom A (1991) The decision to treat by surgery, PTA or conservative methods. Crit Ischaem 1(4):21–26

36. Eklund AE, Eriksson G, Olsson AG (1982) A controlled study showing significant short term effect of PGE_1 in healing of ischaemic ulcers of the lower limb in man. Prostaglandins Leukot Med 8:265–271

37. European Consensus on Critical Limb Ischaemia (1989) Lancet; April 1:737–738

38. Fiessinger JN, Schäfer M (1990) Trial of iloprost versus aspirin treatment for critical limb ischaemia of thromboangitis obliterans. Lancet 335:555–557

39. FitzGerald GA, Smith B, Pederson AK, Brash AR (1984) Increased prostacyclin biosynthesis in patients with severe atherosclerosis and platelet activation. N Engl J Med 310:1065–1068

40. Fonseca V, Dandona P (1990) Treatment of ischaemic ulceration or rest pain with intravenous iloprost: a double-blind placebo controlled study. British Diabetic Association, Glasgow; March 22–24

41. Friedman GD, Klatsky AL, Siegelaub AB (1974) The leukocyte count as a predictor of myocardial infarction. N Engl J Med 290:1275–1278

42. Gallus AS (1986) The use of antithrombotic drugs in artery disease. Clin Haematol 15:509–559

43. Galt SW, McDaniel MD, Ault KA, Mitchell J, Cronenwett JL (1991) Flow cytometric assessment of platelet function in patients with peripheral arterial occlusive disease. J Vasc Surg 14(6):749–755

44. Genton E, Clagett GP, Salzman EW (1986) Antithrombotic therapy in peripheral vascular disease. Arch Int Med 146:470–471

45. Graor RA, Risius B, Young JR, Greisinger MA, Zeich MG (1984) Low dose streptokinase for selective thrombolysis: systemic effects and complications. Radiology 152:35–39

46. Groth CG, Lofström E (1966) The effect of infused high and low molecular weight dextrans on tissue oxygen tension. An experimental study on the rabbit. Acta Chirurgica Scandinavica 31:275 – 289

47. Guilmot J-L, Diot E (1991) Treatment of lower limb ischaemia due to atherosclerosis in diabetic and nondiabetic patients with iloprost, a stable analogue of prostacyclin: Results of a French multicenter trial. Drug Invest 3(5):351 – 359

48. Hickman P, Harrison DK, Hill A, McLaren M, Tamei H, McCollum P, Belch JJF: Exercise in patients with intermittent claudication results in the generation of oxygen derived free radicals and endothelial damage. Oxygen Transport (in press)

49. Hossman V, Auel H, Schhrör K (1986) Placebo-controlled, cross-over study on the action of Iloprost (ZK 36374) in advanced stages of arterial occlusive disease. Trubestein G (ed) In: Conservative Therapy of Arterial Occlusive Disease 186 – 191

50. Iniquez RA, Macaya MC, Hernandez AR, Casaso LJ, Alfonso MF, Giocolea RJ, Zarco GP (1991) The effects of ticlopidine administration at low doses on the incidence of restenosis following percutaneous transluminal coronary angioplasty. Rev Esp Cardiol 44(6):366 – 374

51. Janzon L, Bergist D, Boberg J et al (1990) Prevention of myocardial infarction and stroke in patients with intermittent claudication: effects of ticlopidine. Results from STIMS, the Swedish Ticlopidine Multicentre Study. J Int Med 227:301 – 308

52. Jennings PE, McLaren M, Scott N, Saniabadi A, Belch JJF (1991) The relationship of oxidative stress to thrombotic tendency in type 1 diabetic patients with retinopathy. Diabetic Med 8:860 – 865

53. Jogestrand T, Olsson AG (1985) The effect of intravenous prostaglandin E_1 on ischemic pain and on leg blood-flow in subjects with peripheral artery disease: a double-blind controlled study. Clin Physiol 5:495 – 502

54. Kannel WB, McGee DL (1979) Diabetes and cardiovascular disease: The Framingham Study. JAMA 241:2035 – 2038

55. Kerin MJ, Bavor AID, Greenstein D, Kester RC (1991) Nonsurgical management of peripheral vascular disease. Hospital Update; 873 – 889

56. Kiesewetter H, Jung F, Erdlenbruch W, Wenzel E (1992) Haemodilution in patients with peripheral arterial occlusive disease. Int Angiol 11(3):169 – 175

57. Lau CS, Scott N, Brown JE, Shaw W, Belch JJF (1991) Increased activity of oxygen free radicals during reperfusion in patients undergoing percutaneous peripheral artery balloon angioplasty. Int Angiol 10(4):244 – 246

58. Lowe GDO, Dunlop DJ, Lawson DH, Pollock JG, Watt JK, Forbes CD, Prentice CRM, Drummond MM (1982) Double-blind controlled clinical trial of ancrod for ischemic rest pain of the leg. Angiology 33(1):46 – 50

59. Lowe GPO (1990) Pathophysiology of critical limb ischaemia. In: Dormandy J, Stock G (eds) Critical Leg Ischaemia – Its Pathophysiology nad Management. Springer, Heidelberg 17:40

60. McCollum CN, Alexander C, Kenchington G et al (1991) Antiplatelet drugs in femoropopliteal vein bypasses. A multicentre trial. J Vasc Surg 13:150 – 162

61. McNamara TO, Fischer JR (1985) Thrombolysis of peripheral arterial and graft occlusions: improved results using high dose urokinase. Am J Roentgenol 144:769 – 775

62. Meehan SE, Preece PE, Walker WF (1982) The usefulness of naftidrofuryl in severe peripheral ischaemia – a symptomatic assessment using linear analogue scales. Angiology 33(10): 625 – 634

63. Murray RR, Helves RC, White RI (1987) Long segment femoropopliteal stenoses in angioplasty, a boon or a bust? Radiology 162:473 – 476

64. Negus D, Irving JD, Friedgood A (1985) Intraarterial prostacyclin compared to praxilene in the management of advanced atherosclerotic lower limb ischaemia. In: Gryglewski R, Szczeklik A, McGiff JC (eds) Prostacyclin. Clinical Trials. New York: Raven Press 107:119

65. Nizankowski R, Krolikowski W, Bielatowicz J, Szczeklik A (1985) Prostacyclin for ischemic ulcers in peripheral arterial disease. A random assignment, placebo controlled study. Thrombos Res 37:21 – 28

66. Noda K (1986) Study on one-shot intravenous administration method of lipo PGE_1, on diabetic neuropathy. Jap J Clin Exper Med 63(a):305 – 308

67. Norgren L, Alwmark A, Angqvist KA, Hedberg B, Bergqvist D (1990) A stable prostacyclin analogue, iloprost, in the treatment of ischaemic ulcers of the lower limb. A Scandinavian-Polish placebo controlled, randomised multicenter study. Eur J Vasc Surg 4:463−467

68. O'Riordain DS, O'Donnell JA (1991) Realistic expectations for the patient with intermittent claudication. Br J Surg 78:861−863

69. Oberender H, Krais Th, Schäfer M, Belcher G (1989) Clinical benefits of iloprost, a stable prostacyclin (PGI_2) analog, in severe peripheral arterial disease (PAD). In: Advances in Prostaglandin, Thromboxane and Leukotriene Research. Samuelsson B, Wong P Y-K, Sunn FF (eds) Raven Press Ltd, New York; Vol 19

70. Prevention of coronary heart disease: scientific background and new clinical guidelines (1993) Recommendations of the European Atherosclerosis Society prepared by the International Task Force for prevention of Coronary Heart Disease. Nutrition, Metabolism and Cardiovascular Disease 2:113−156

71. Ricotta JJ, Green RM, DeWeese JA (1987) Use and limitations of thrombolytic therapy in the treatment of peripheral arterial ischaemia: results of a multi-institutional questionnaire. J Vasc Surg 6:46−50

72. Rowley MR, Ray SA, Loh A, Talbot SA; Dormandy JA, Bevan DH (1993) Acquired hypercoagulable states and occlusion of surgical revascularization procedures in peripheral arterial disease. Thromb Haemostas 69(6):1204

73. Schuler JJ, Flanigan DP, Holcraft JW, Ursprung KK, Mohrland JS, Pyke E (1984) Efficacy of prostaglandin E_1 in the treatment of lower extremity ischaemic ulcers secondary to peripheral vascular occlusive disease. J Vasc Surg 1:160−170

74. Shaw SWJ, Johnson RH (1975) The effect of naftidrofuryl on the metabolic response to exercise in man. Acta Neurol Scand 52:231−237

75. Shearman C, Smith F, Hickey N, Simms MH (1993) Pharmacological Augmentation of Arterial Reconstruction in CLI. Crit Ischaem 3:51−55

76. Sonecha TN, Nicolaides AN (1991) The relationship between intermittent claudication and coronary artery disease − is it more than we think? Vasc Med Rev 2(2):137−146

77. Szczeklik A, Skawinski S, Gluszko P, Nizankowski R, Szczeklik J, Gryglewski RJ (1979) Successful therapy of advances arteriosclerosis obliterans with prostacyclin. Lancet, May 26:1111−1114

78. Taggart I, Wishart GS, Cuschieri RJ, MacBain GC (1989) Effect of intravenous naftidrofuryl on transcutaneous oxygen pressure in severe peripheral vascular disease. Angiology 69:895−898

79. Telles GC, Campbell WB, Wood RF, Collin J, Baird RN, Morris PJ (1984) Prostaglandin E_1 in severe lower limb ischaemia: a double-blind controlled trial. Br J Surg 71:506−508

80. The Second European Consensus Document on Chronic Critical Leg Ischaemia (1992) Antiplatelet drugs in critical leg ischaemia. Critical Ischaemia 2(3):26−29

81. Trübestein G, Ludwig M, Diehm C, Gruss JD, Horsch S (1987) Prostaglandin E_1 bei arterieller Verschlußkrankheit im Stadium III und IV. Ergebnisse einer multizentrischen Studie. Dtsch Med Wochenschr 112:955−959

82. Trübestein G, von Bary S, Breddin K et al (1989) Intravenous prostagladin E_1 versus pentoxifylline therapy in chronic arterial occlusive disease − a controlled randomized multicenter study. VASA 28:44−49

83. Utsunomiya T, Kransz MM, Valeri CR, Shepro D, Hecktman HB (1980) Treatment of pulmonary embolism with prostacyclin. Surgery 88:25−30

84. Verhaeghe R (1991) Prophylactic antiplatelet therapy in peripheral arterial disease. Drugs 42 (Suppl 5):51−57

85. Verhaeghe R, Bounameaux H (1991) Peripheral arterial occlusion: thromboembolism and antithrombotic therapy. In: Fuster V, Verstraete M (eds) Thrombosis in Cardiovascular Disorders. Philadelphia: WB Saunders Company, 423−449

86. Vreeken J, van Aken WG (1971) Spontaneous aggregation of blood platelets as a cause of idiopathic thrombosis and recurrent painful toes and fingers. Lancet 2:1394−1397

87. Wiseman S, Kenchington G, Dain R, Marshall CE, McCollum CN, Greenhalgh RM, Powell JT (1989) Influence of smoking and plasma factors on patency of femoropopliteal vein grafts. Brit Med J 299:643−646

88. Yonda T (1986) The effects of bolus injection of lipo PGE_1, on ischaemic peripheral arterial disease in humans. Cardioangiol 20(2):159−167

89. Zahavi J, Zahavi M (1985) Enhanced platelet release reaction, shortened platelet survival time and increased platelet aggregation and plasma thromboxane B_2 in chronic obstructive arterial disease. Thromb Haemostas 53:105–109

Authors' address:

Dr. J. J. F. Belch MD FRCP
Reader and Consultant Physician
Head of Section of Vascular Medicine

Mr. P. McCollum FRCS
Consultant Vascular Surgery
Director of the Vascular Laboratory and Surgery
University Department of Medicine
Ninewells Hospital and Medical School
Dundee DD1 9SY
Scotland

Limb salvage, vascular procedures versus primary amputation

K. Balzer

Gefäßchirurgische Klinik des Evangelischen Krankenhauses
Mülheim an der Ruhr, Chefarzt Dr. Balzer, FRG

Vascular surgery made a lot of progress, especially in the last 15 years. The patency rate of bifurcated grafts 5 years after implantation is more than 80%.

The results of the autologues venous bypass in femoral artery occlusions are, with 70%, almost as good. The use of alloplastic grafts reduces the patency rates by 10% in the popliteal position. Crural reconstructions show a tendency towards worse results, and even worse outcome can be seen in the pedal area (Fig. 1).

Other risk factors of arteriosclerosis also worsen the prognosis. In our experience, the limb salvage rate in patients with diabetic gangrene falls under 40% 2 years after reconstruction. A high proportion of patients with critical leg ischemia have coexisting diseases such as cardiovascular and renal disorders which may render them unsuitable for general anesthesia or surgery. Whether or not the patient is fit to undergo surgery depends on the extent to which other organs have been affected by the underlying atherosclerotic disease, the patient's age, concomitant risk factors, and past diseases.

The feasibility of a surgical reconstruction must be confirmed by angiography. The success of surgery depends, as outlined before, on the level of the obstruction; in general, the more distal the obstruction, the worse the prognosis.

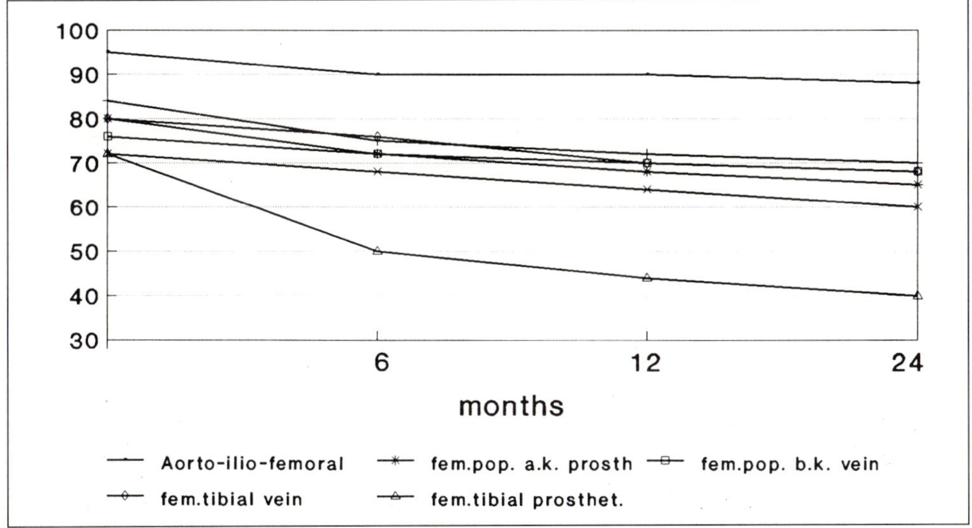

Fig. 1. Patency rates. Vascular surgical procedures

The risk of, and increased cost associated with, a failed bypass procedure must be borne in mind when deciding which alternative to take. Early graft failure (< 30 days) may be due to incorrect choice of operation, operative technique, poor distal run-off, low flow through the graft or graft surface thrombogenicity. Late failure graft (> 30 days) is usually caused by thrombosis, intimal hyperplasia, progressive atherosclerosis or graft structure abnormalities. Smoking and high fibrinogen levels play a part in late graft failures. If the procedure fails there could be an increased risk of mortality when further major surgery is needed for amputation as documented in some literature. There is always a problem in deciding whether reconstructive surgery is a risk worth taking. It is important to weigh the risk/benefit ratio. In cases where limb salvage apperas to be virtually impossible, primary amputation should be considered.

Risk of amputation

Amputation is the most serious from of intervention. Because of the better prognosis for rehabilitation and the lower mortality rate (8% versus 18%) below-knee amputation is preferable to above-knee amputation. Amputees have a very poor prognosis: approximately 40% will die within 2 years because of the interaction of arteriosclerotic and coronary artery disease, only 70% of below-knee amputations heal primarily, 15% heal by secondary intervention, and 15% require an above-knee amputation after a failed below-knee amputation. Full mobility is only achieved in 50% and 25% of below-knee and above-knee amputees, respectively (Table 1, Fig. 2).

Possibility and risk of reconstructive surgery

Until the advent of angioplasty and other reopening procedures, surgical reconstruction was the only method available for directly treating the underlying atherosclerosis in the large vessels. It is still the most commonly used form of treatment for critical leg ischemia. The aim of such surgery is to bypass of remove the stenosed or occluded artery segment.

The main methods employed by the vascular surgeon are as follows:

Endarterectomy: With this method the occluding plaque is cut out of the artery. In some cases an autologous vein or synthetic patch is stitched in to widen the lumen of the artery.

Bypass surgery: This operation involves the bridging of the stenosed or occluded vascular segment with a venous transplant from the patient, or using synthetic

Table 1. Risk of amputation

	below knee	above knee
Hospital-mortality	4%	8%
1 year mortality	8%	20%
primary healing	70%	85%
secondary healing	15%	12%
further amputation	15%	3%
full mobility	50%	25%

114

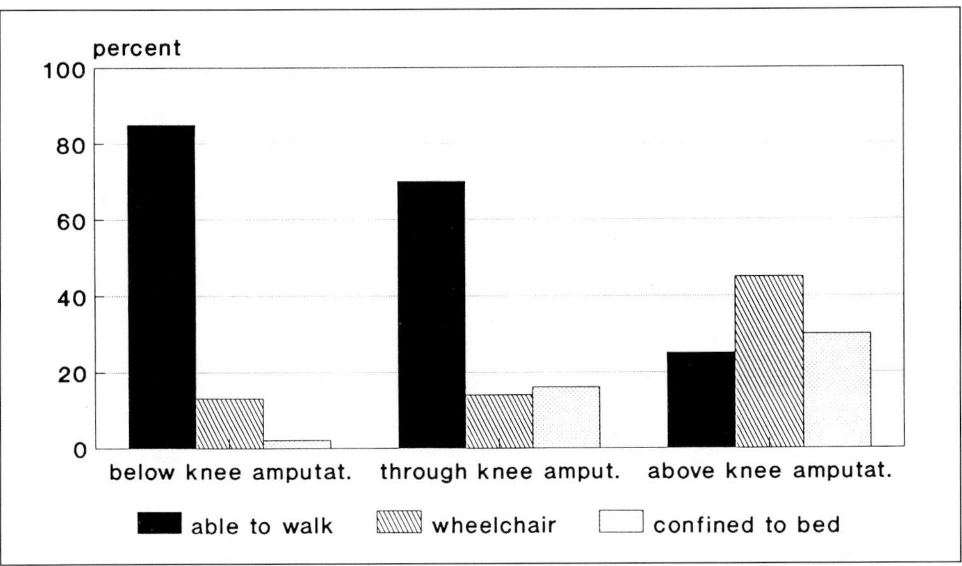

Fig. 2. Degree of rehabilitation according to site of amputation

prostheses if no autologous material is available. Critical leg ischemia is often caused by disease occurring at several levels, and this often requires combined procedures. The patency rates of reconstructive procedures were shown before. Frequent assessment of graft patency and immediate treatment of potential problems is preferable to trying to rectify a graft failure. More than 20% of autologous vein grafts fail because of strictures in the first year. These stenoses should be treated by angioplasty or surgery and not be allowed to progress to complete occlusion. Various objective measurements are available to detect stenoses which could progress to occlusions such as post-exercise ankle pressure measurement, duplex scanning, digital substraction angiography, and impedance measurement.

Surgical procedures versus primary amputation

A succesful operation does not solve the problem of the progressive basic disease. A number of patients cannot be operated successfully because of the multiple peripheral occlusions, especially in case of diabetes. Sometimes the multimorbidity does not allow a vascular surgical procedure. Vascular surgery or interventional techniques are the methods of first choice in any patient with critical limb ischemia. But there are a lot of patients who have already been operated which makes another vascular reconstruction impossible. The patency rates show the statistical success of vascular surgical operations. But what happens to the unsuccessfully operated patients or to the re-occluded bypass procedures? In these cases a therapy with prostaglindines or the spinal cord stimulation may be discussed. Of course, there is a number of patient in which, because of extended gangrene, unhealed limited amputations can be considered hopeless for any further treatment; recommendation 25 of the critical ischemia consensus document states that "primary amputation should only be undertaken if the possibility of revascularization procedures has been excluded". In practice, revascularization might be rejected because it is deemed to be inappropriate, unsafe, impossible or inadvisable. In these cases by treatment by medication as well is usually impossible. Harris and Moody summarized some reasons for rejecting attempts at revascularization:

1) Reconstruction inappropriate: Necrosis of a major part of the limb. Functionally useless limb.

2) Reconstruction unsafe: Life threatening toxemia from ischemic tissue.

3) Reconstruction impossible: Complete absence of operable distal vessels.

4) Reconstruction inadvisable: Patent distal vessels and revascularization technically possible, but with poor chance of success.

The working group for critical limb ischemia made the observation that "in some cases primary amputation may be better than subjecting the patient to repeated surgical procedures with little chance of success and increasing mortality and morbidity." This can be a very difficult decision and a team approach may be very useful. Each case should therefore be assessed on its individual merit and every patient should have a chance for vascular surgical reconstruction. The most difficult situation to judge to the patient's best advantage is that in which surgical reconstruction may be technically possible, but with a pure chance of lasting success. This most often occurs when occlusive disease extends into the infracrural vessels, as is often the case in those with critical ischemia. Although bypass grafts to the ankle and foot are now commonplace, some of these operations approach the limits of surgical effi-

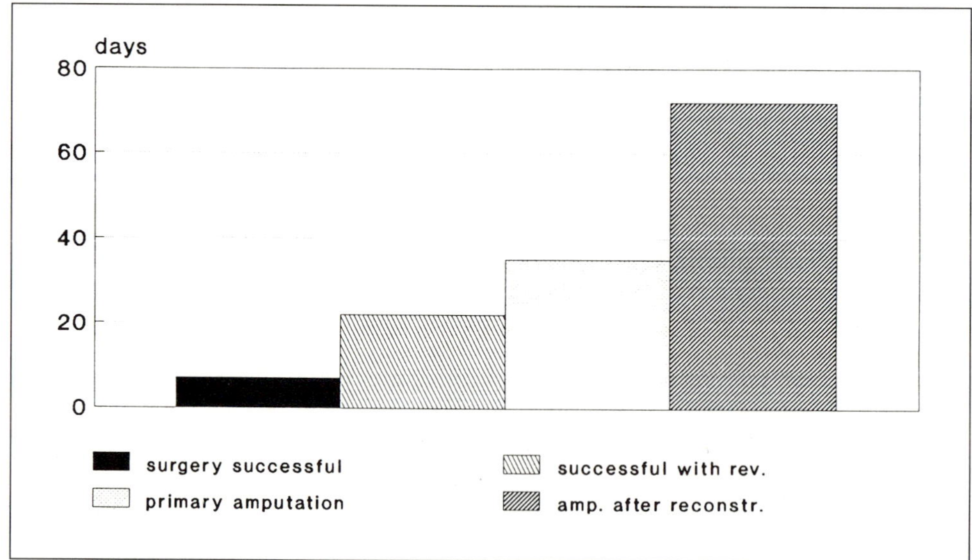

Fig. 3. Time of hospitalization after operation

116

cacy. Autologous vein grafts from groin to ankle provide at least a chance of limb salvage and are indicated wherever possible but the results using synthetic grafts fall considerably short with patency rates of only 25 – 30% after 1 year. If a long bypass is indicated and there is not sufficient autologous vein it has to be decided whether to attempt reconstruction or to advise primary amputation. It has to be stated that there is no adequate measure of success. So recommendations are not possible and a more flexible approach is required. But the decision has to be made, which procedure is going to be the last chance before amputation. This way no further revision is necessary.

Until now, it has been impossible to predict the possibility of vascular reconstruction using different kinds of measurements, such as TPO2, thermography, laser Doppler, peripheral resistance, radio-isotope measurements and, of course, angiography.

The duration of hospitalization can be a sign for a satisfactory therapy. In our hospital, we have the shortest time after successful vascular surgical or interventional therapy (7.2 days). After re-occluded but successfully re-opened vascular procedures the time of hospitalization increases rapidly (22 days). Primary amputation requires, on average, a hospitalization of 35 days, amputation of the unsuccessfully operated patient requires more than 2 months (Fig. 3). Mortality rate increases with the length of the stay in the hospital. It is below 1% in the first group and increases to 8% in the group with primary amputation. But it is lower in patients after vascular surgical reconstruction. This means that in our experience these operations do not increase the risk, as claimed in some publications. Erasmi found that more than 2 reoperations did not bring more success. However the mortality rate after 3 operations increased significantly, that is up to 50%. May be that better physiotherapy will reduce the risk to that today we have a "normal" risk of amputation either in patients with or without vascular surgery. But the costs are tremendous so that in cases with only very little chance of success primary amputation is the method of choice (Fig. 4,5).

Patient's requiring below-knee or above-knee amputations are not directly comparable and the difference in mortality cannot be attributed solely to the level of theamputation. The main advantage of the below-knee procedure is the preservation of the natural knee joint, This can certainly make an enormous difference in the degree of mobility which patients achieve following fitting of a prosthesis. If limb salvage or minor amputation is not possible the below knee or through knee amputation is to be considered a success of the vascular surgical procedure as compared to the primary above-knee amputation. Shifting the amputation wounds distally as better healing process following amputation is caused by the improved arterial circulation.

For the bad prognosis of amputation the consensus document on critical limb ischemia states in its recommendation 21: *A reconstructive procedure should be attempted so long as there is a reasonable chance of saving a useful limb in a patient with evidence of sufficient run-off and [who] is fit for surgery.* A graft failure may be related to the flow properties of blood through the vessel. Greater graft length increases the occlusion rate, increased diameter decreases the flow velocity, and increases the occlusion rate. There is a higher incidence of graft failure with prosthetic materials than with autologous vein graft. But graft patency is not necessarily equivalent to limb salvage. With time there is a greater discrepancy between graft patency and limb salvage due to collateral formation. Late graft failure may not affect the viability of the leg. Amputition is required more frequently for early than for late

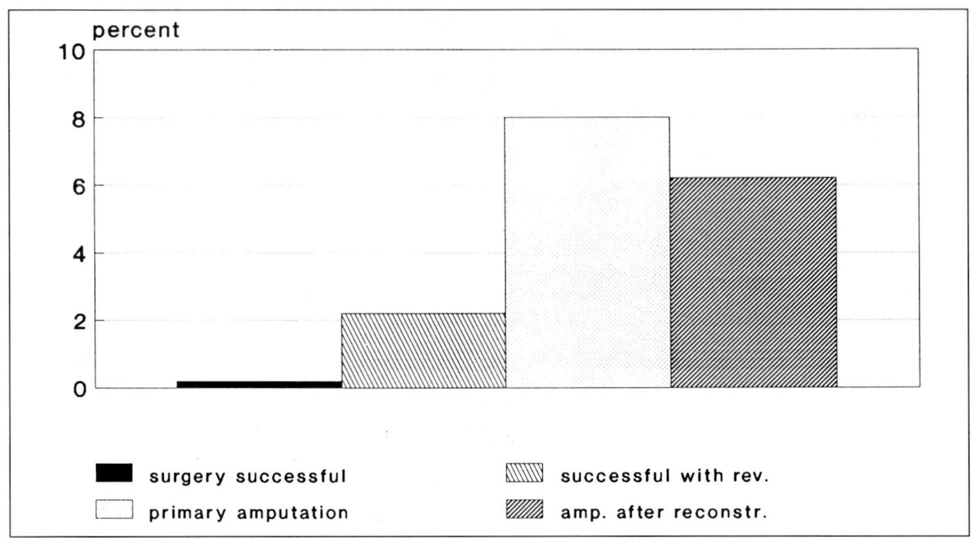

Fig. 4. Hospital-Mortality after operation

graft failures. Thus, the longer a graft stays open the lower the likelihood of amputation.

Natural history of POAD

Two case histories are useful as examples:

1) First, a 46-year-old male whose femoral artery stenosis was treated with angioplasty twice and who was subsequently operated three times in the femoral and popliteal region: All of these procedures could be considered successful only for a short period of time. He again suffered from an extended necrosis and the angiogram shows occlusions of all arteries of the left lower limb. It was necessary to perform a composite pedal bypass procedure from the femoral to the anterior tibial artery and from there to the posterior tibial artery. The bypass worked for 3 days only. A thrombectomy and a-v-fistula were performed. After a renewed occlusion and thrombectomy a catheter for regional thrombolysis was implanted. The bypass could be re-opened in this way, but worked for 6 months only, whereas necrosis healed completely. At this time, restpain reoccurred. Because a surgical procedure was not possible anymore, the patient was treated with PGE_1. The rest pain disappeared for 3 months. After that it was necessary to amputate the left limb above-knee because of enxtensive gangrene. The history of the right leg was similar and he lost it 2 years later. Two months after the second amputation he died because of ischemic heart failure.
2) A 76-year-old female was operated successfully with a crural PTFE bypass procedure to the only open anterior tibial artery. It remains patent until today, which is 5 years after reconstruction.

118

As shown in these examples it is impossible to predict the natural history of POAD. Only the age of the patient seems to be a safe predictive value: The younger the patient with POAD the worse the prognosis. But the younger the patient, the more surgical treatment for limb salvage is required.

Summary

Recommendation for primary amputation is summarized in the following (after Harris and Moody, modified):

1) Primary amputation should only be undertaken if the possibility of revascularization procedures has been excluded.
2) Angiography should always be performed before major amputation in patients with potentially reversible critical ischemia. In case of doubt, an angiogram should be performed during operation after exposure of the below knee arteries.
3) Prosthetic grafts to the ankle rarely succeed. However, they might still be indicated as an alternative to amputation.
4) In some cases primary amputation may be better than subjecting the patient to repeated surgical procedures with little chance of success and increasing mortality and morbidity.
5) Below-knee amputation is preferred to above-knee because of lower morbidity and mortality rates and better mobility following operation.
6) Below-knee amputation is considered successful after vascular surgery.
7) Objective measurements of skin perfusion should be employed to aid the selection of the level of amputation wherever possible. At present, there is still no valid measurement for predicting the success of vascular surgery operations.
8) Amputations should be followed by appropriate rehabilitation.

References

1. Adamek L, Balzer K (1988) Stellenwert und Ergebnisse peripherer gefäßchirurgisch-rekonstruktiver Maßnahmen in der Behandlung der AVK beim Diabetiker. angio 10, 5:227–231
2. Ascer E, Veuth FJ, Morris L, Lesser ML, Gupta SK, Samson RH, Scher VA, White Flores SA (1984) Components of outlow resistance and their correlation with graft patency of lower extremity arterial reconstructions. J Vasc Surg 1:817–828
3. Beard JD, Scott DJ, Evans JM, Skidmore R, Horrocks M (1988) Pulse generated run-off, a new method of determining calf vessel patency. Br J Surg 74 (4):361–363
4. Bell PRF, Charlesworth D, De Palma R, Jamieson C (1982) The definition of critical ischaemia of a limb. Br J Surg 69:52, 1
5. Charles D (1987) Problems related to run in and run off with reference to the profundafemoris artery and secondary femoropopliteal bypass. Acta Chir Scand 538–543
6. Cross FW, Cotton LT (1985) Chemical lumbar sympathectomy for ischaemic rest pain. Am J Surg 150:341–345
7. Daling RC, Linton RR (1972) Durability of femoropopliteal reconstructions. Am J Surg 123:472–547
8. Dardik H, Kahn M, Dardik I, Sussmann B, Ibrahim IM (1982) Influence of failed vascular bypass procedures on vonversionof below knee to above knee amputation levels. Surgery 91:64–69

 9. De Weese JA, Rob CG (1978) Effect of arterial reconstruction on limb salvage: A ten year appraisal. Arch Surg 113:1297–1304

10. Dormandy JA, Mahir MS (1986) The natural history of peripheral atheromatous disease of the legs. In: Greenhalgh RM, Jamieson CW, Nicolaides AN (eds) Vascular surgery: Issues in Current Practice. Grune and Stratton, London, pp 3–19

11. Dormandy JA, Stock G (1990) Critical leg ischaemia. Springer Berlin Heidelberg New York

12. Dormandy JA, Thomas PRS (1988) What is the natural history of critically ischaemic patient with and without his leg? In: Greenhalgh RM, Jamieson CW, Nicolaides AN (eds) Limb salvage and amputation for vascular disease. Publ Saunders, pp 11–26

13. Evans LE, Webster MW, Brooks DH, Bahnson HT (1980) Pheriperal-arterial surgery. N Engl J Med 302:491–503

14. Gardener GA Jr, Harrington DP, Kolrun W, Whittemore A, Mannick JA, Levin DC (1987) Salvage of occluded arterial bypass grafts by means of thrombolysis. J Vasc Surg 9:426–432

15. Gupta SK, Veith FJ (1980) Below-knee bypass for limb salvage: Comparison of autogenous saphenous vein, polytetrafluorethylene and composite Dacron-autogenous-vein grafts. Arch Surg 115:833–837

16. Gupta SK, Veith FJ, Ascer E, White Flores SA, Gleedmann ML (1988) Cost factors inlimb threatening ischaemia due to infrainguinal artherosclerosis. European J Vasc Surg 2:151–155

17. Harris PL, Read F, Eardley A, Charlesworth D, Wakefield J, Sellwood RA (1974) The fate of elderly amputees. Br J Surg 61:665–668

18. Harris PL, Campbell H (1986) Femoro-distal bypass for critical ischaemia: is the use of prosthetic grafts justified? Ann Vasc Surg 1:66–72

19. Harris P, Moody P (1990) Amputations. In: Dormandy A, Stock G (eds) Critical leg ischaemia. Springer Berlin Heidelberg New York

20. Hertzer NR (1980) Three years experience with expanded polytetrafluorethylene artrial grafts for limb salvage. Amer J Surg 104:214

21. Hobson RW, O'Donnell JA, Jamil Z, Mehta K (1981) Why do reported graft patency rates vary so wide? In: Greenhalgh RM (ed) Femoro-distal bypass. Pittmann, London

22. Holstein P (1985) Skin perfusion pressure measured by radioisotope washout for predicting wound healing in lower limb amputation for arterial occlusive disease. Thesis Acta Orthop Scand Suppl 213

23. Johnson WC (1977) Autogenous venous grafts ten years later. Surgery 82:775–784

24. Parvin SD, Evens DH, Bell PRF (1985) Peripheral resistance measurement in the assessment of severe peripheral vascular disease. Br J Surg 72:751–753

25. Ratcliff DA, Clyne CAC, Chant ADB, Webster JHH (1984) Prediction of amputation wound healing: the role of transcutaneous oxygen tension in the selection of amputation level. Am J Surg 147:510–517

26. Seibel RMM, Carstensen G, Balzer K, Grönemeyer DHW, Sehnert C (1989) CT-gesteuerte lumbale Symphatikusausschaltung bei der Behandlung der peripheren arteriellen Verschlußkrankheit (AVK). In: Grönemeyer DHW, Seibel RMM (eds) Interventionelle Computertomographie. Ueberreuter Wissenschaft, Wien Berlin

27. Simms MH (1988) Is pedal arch patency a pre-requisite for successful reconstruction? In: Greenhalgh RM, Jamieson CW, Nicolaides AN (eds) Limb Salvage and Amputation for Vascular Disease. Publ Saunders, London, pp 49–62

28. Spence VA, Walker WF, Troup IM, Murdoch G (1981) Amputation of the ischaemic limb: selection of the optimum site by thermography. Angiology 32:155–169

29. Szilagyi DE, Hagemann JA, Smith RF, Elliott JP (1985) Femoropopliteailer Bypass: Autologe Vene oder PTFE-Prothese? Angio 7, 1:13–20

30. Stockel M, Oresen J, Bröchner-Mortensen J, Emnius H (1982) Standardised photoelectric technique as routine method for selection of amputation level. Acta Orthop Scand 53:875

31. Stockmann U Pidda (1983) Ein Novum in der cruralen Gefäßchirurgie. Angio 5, 2:67–71

32. Tuchmann A, Strasser K, Axenkopf G (1972) Obliterationsgrad proximaler Unterschenkelarterien in Beziehung zum Ergebnis femoro-poplitealer Thrombendarteriektomien. Vasa 1:256

33. Veith FJ, Moss CM, Fell SC, Rhodes BA, Haimovici H (1981) Femoropopliteal bypass to the isolated popliteal segment: is PTFE graft acceptable? Surgery 89:296

34. Wilson SE, Wolf GL, Cross A (1989) Percutaneous transluminal angioplasty versus operation
    for peripheral arteriosclerosis. Report of a randomised trial in a selected group of patients.
    J Vasc Surg 9:1−9
35. Wolfe JHN (1988) Critical ischaemia − is this concept of value? In: Greenhalgh RW, Jamieson
    CW, Nicolaides AN (eds) Limb Salvage and Amputation for Vascular Disease. WB Saunders,
    London, pp 3−10

Anschrift des Verfassers:

Dr. Klaus Balzer
Gefäßchirurgische Klinik
Evang. Krankenhaus
Wertgasse 30
D-45468 Mülheim an der Ruhr
FRG

Assessment of the microcirculation

Evaluation of the skin microcirculation by photoplethysmography, laser Doppler velocimetry, and transcutaneous measurements of pO_2

J. D. Blankensteijn and W. M. Abbott

Division of Vascular Surgery, Department of Surgery,
Massachusetts General Hospital, Harvard Medical School, Boston, USA

Introduction

Treatment of peripheral arterial occlusive disease (PAOD) should be directed at the associated dysfunction of the target tissues. In patients with lower limb ischemia, conditions become critical when blood supply no longer meets the metabolic demands, typically of the acral skin.

When treating symptoms of vascular disease, an objective estimate of the severity of the disease is essential. Judgements to be made include the potential effectiveness of vascular reconstructions, the skin healing capacity, and the selection of amputation level. History and physical examination frequently fail to provide an accurate assessment in this respect. So, clinical staging of patients with PAOD is commonly based on evaluation of hemodynamic and anatomic changes in the "macrocirculation", even though the skin is the actual target tissue.

The skin microcirculation is the circulation in small arterioles (< 300 μm), capillaries and venules. The most important function of the skin microcirculation is tissue nutrition, although it is also involved in regulation of blood pressure, homeostasis of interstitial fluids, and thermoregulation [1].

Because of the sigmoidal character of the hemoglobin binding curve for oxygen, normal tissue metabolism can be maintained even when arterial pressure and flow are substantially diminished. For this reason direct evaluation of the skin microcirculation cannot be an accurate measure of milder stages of PAOD.

The above mentioned objectives of vascular investigations, however, together with the frequent presence of added micro-vessel disease (diabetes mellitus) in PAOD have led to increasing interest in the microcirculation of the skin. Since the late 1970s, several new noninvasive techniques to evaluate skin microcirculation have emerged [15]. In this review, the current status of three methods is described: photoplethysmography (PPG), transcutaneous measurement of partial oxygen pressure ($tcpO_2$), and laser Doppler velocimetry (LDV). In order to better understand the nature of the physiologic parameters these methods provide and to demonstrate why one test may be more appropriate than another in certain pathologic conditions, an update on skin microcirculatory anatomy and physiology is presented first.

Anatomy and physiology of skin microcirculation

In the dermis an upper and a lower horizontal plexus of arterioles and venules can be identified. The lower horizontal plexus is formed by perforating vessels from the underlying muscles and subcutaneous fat, at the dermal-subcutaneous interface. From this plexus arterioles and venules form direct connections with the upper horizontal plexus as well as provide lateral tributaries to hair bulbs and sweat glands. The upper horizontal network is found in the papillary dermis and gives rise to the capillary loops of the dermal papillae. Here, 1 to 2 mm below the epidermal surface, the bulk of the microcirculation resides [2].

The capillary loop arises from a terminal arteriole in the upper horizontal network, it is composed of an ascending limb, an intrapapillary loop having a hairpin turn, and a descending limb which connects with a postcapillary venule in the horizontal plexus. The intrapapillary arterial loop abruptly develops venous characteristics after the vessel leaves the dermal papilla [4]. Very few capillary loops have sphincters. Still, this function is maintained by endothelial cells bulging in the lumen at the junctions of capillaries and postcapillary venules (pseudocontractility) [21].

Within the horizontal plexus, arteriolar-rich and relatively avascular zones are found, resembling a "micro-livedo" pattern [3]. Furthermore, a rhythmical variation in arteriole diameter and blood flow called vasomotion has been recognized [30].

There appear to be two classes of microvessels in the skin, one responsible primarily for tissue perfusion and one responsible primarily for thermoregulation [3]. Less than 10% of the total skin blood flow passes through the capillary loops of the dermal papillae for skin nutrition. The remaining 90% passes directly into the venules of the upper horizontal network through the arteriovenous shunts [1]. These AV-shunts are not merely AV-channels but have an intricate structure, similar to renal glomeruli. They are therefore thought to have specific function for body temperature-control.

Skin blood flow is regulated by neural factors, hormones, factors released from endothelial cells and autoregulatory mechanisms. Recently, several aspects of the local regulatory mechanisms and their interactions with neural factors have been elucidated. Historically, however, most attention has been given to the role of autonomic neurons, especially the sympathetic vasoconstrictor neurons. Parasympathetic innervation is generally considered absent in the skin [23].

The arteriolar segment is encompassed in a sleeve of smooth muscle cells innervated by sympathetic nerve fibers [2]. The sympathetic (adrenergic) nerve system produced noradrenalin, which has effect on spiral muscle in arteries, arterioles, AV-shunts and venules. Capillaries are not under sympathetic control. They react passively to changes in afferent and efferent vessels and to local metabolic conditions. Sweat-glands, innervated by sympathetic neurons, can also produce large quantities of bradykinin, decreasing vasoconstrictive tone.

The microcirculation of most regions (except hand and foot) are controlled by an increase or decrease in venoconstrictive tone, controlled by sympathetic innervation. Hand and foot are mostly controlled by arterioconstriction, predominantly of arteriovenous shunts [23]. However, even after blockade of cholinergic and noradrenergic transmission, blood vessels can be actively dilated in response to nerve stimulation [13].

Several neuropeptides, including substance P (SP) and calcitonin gene-related peptide (CGRP), have been identified in nerve fibers innervating small arteries, arterioles, and capillaries. Antidromic stimulation of dorsal roots leads to release of these neuropeptides that share a strong vasodilatory effect. The vascular endothelium and its autacoid nitric oxide play an important role in setting vascular tone according to the physiological needs of the skin. This vasodilator system appears to be an impor-

126

tant target of afferent nerve-derived vasoactive peptides. The afferent vasodilator neurons are also interacting with the sympathetic vasoconstrictor neurons, and the neuropeptides are capable of activating mast cells to release histamine and other vasodilatory factors. Even intravascular leucocytes can be activated by neuropeptides, resulting in the release of prostaglandin, thromboxane and cytokine mediators [13]. These recent findings shed new light on the concept of "neurogenic inflammation".

In addition, a so-called sensory axon reflex exists by which local stimuli ("local red reaction") can cause regional vasodilation [21]. A similar sympathetic axon reflex probably also exists [23]. Furthermore, local vasodilation may be induced by anoxic and acidosis or via secretion of histamine, bradykinin, etc.

Techniques

Photoplethysmography (PPG)

Plethysmography measures changes in volume. In most parts of the body these changes are related to changes in blood volume. Strictly speaking, PPG is not true plethysmography, since it does not directly measure volume change. The photoplethysmograph is composed of an infrared light emitting diode and a photo sensor. The degree to which this light is attenuated by the red blood cells is proportional to the quantity of blood present, but the exact origin and meaning of the signal has not been resolved [25].

Relatively transparent anatomic parts such as the ear lobe may be assessed by transillumination, but the same measures may be obtained by the PPG analysis of reflected light.

Because PPG is difficult to calibrate, its use is generally limited to the determination of relative changes during a single application. It may be linked to an alternate current (AC) or direct current (DC) amplifier. In the AC-mode, the pulsatile component of the distal pressure is measured. In the DC-mode, slower changes in cutaneous blood content can be assessed, allowing measurements of blood pressure and venous incompetence.

PPG cannot differentiate between nutritional capillary flow and flow through deeper AV-shunts.

Transcutaneous measurement of partial oxygen pressure (tcpO$_2$)

TcpO$_2$ was originally developed for continuous arterial pO$_2$ monitoring in neonates [14]. In addition, it is now a common procedure in patients receiving intensive care, anesthesia, and artificial ventilation to obtain sufficient permeabillity to gases, the skin needs to be heated to between 43 and 45 °C. The resulting vasodilation under the electrode overrides vasoregulatory vasoconstrictive changes in the skin microcirculation [20]. Through a layer of contact fluid and the epidermis, the electrochemical sensor measures gases transferred from the dermis. An initial period of 15 to 20 min is required for stabilization of skin blood flow before continuous monitoring becomes possible.

In the late 1970s, tcpO$_2$ gained attention as a method to estimate skin oxygenation in patients with PAOD [26]. Since then, numerous reports have evaluated

$tcpO_2$ in staging PAOD, predicting ulcer healing, selecting amputation levels, and measuring pharmacological effects [22].

There is a non-linear (hyperbolic) relationship between $tcpO_2$ and ankle systolic arterial pressures and in vascular patients $tcpO_2$ indirectly reflects skin perfusion rates related to the non-linear part of the flow hyperbola [22]. However, if the intervening tissue consumes all oxygen between the capillary loop and the electrode, oxygen cannot be detected transcutaneously although skin oxygen requirements may still be satisfied. This phenomenon is referred to as the flow-insensitive range of the $tcpO_2$ probe.

Because of the necessary heating of the skin, provocation of vasomotor reflexes (reactive hyperaemia) and vasoactive substances may not cause the same reactions as in the non-heated skin. Leg elevation and dependency and oxygen inhalation have been used successfully to enhance diagnostic sensitivity. With respect to reproductibility, readings may vary 5 to 10 mmHg around the mean $tcpO_2$ values between 10 and 40 mmHg [22]. Cardiopulmonary influences may be eliminated by calculating values normalized to the skin of the chest.

Still, many physiological, methodological, and technical factors influence $tcpO_2$ measurements. Increased age and local edema formation for instance reduce $tcpO_2$ values, and the incidence of these factors is particularly high in the group of patients subjected to $tcpO_2$ assessment.

Laser Doppler Velocimetry (LDV)

The use of LDV to study circulation was first described by Stern in 1975 [24]. The technique is based on the changes in frequency (Doppler effect) and amplitude of low-energy laser-light when it is scattered by moving cells in the vascular bed. Red or near infrared monochromatic light from a low-power laser is directed to the tissue to be studied. The radiation penetrates to a depth of $1-1.5$ mm. The light scattered back from the tissue is collected and analyzed. Because of the way Doppler shifts are measured the system is insensitive to the direction of movement.

In practice, each photon undergoes multiple scattering from many red blood cells and for each scattering event the angle between the incident ray of light and the direction of motion of the red blood and may vary between 0 and 180°. The measured frequency shift is therefore derived from an unknown average value of this angle [25]. AC and DC components are analyzed and an estimate of the relative numbers of cells moving at different velocities, and, hence, total blood flow is provided. The final signal is a function of the product of the velocity and the number of moving particles (flux).

LDV measures much more than capillary circulation. Flow in AV-shunts and subdermal plexuses is also measured. Severe skin ischemia may therefore exist despite high LDV values (in AV-shunts) [16].

The principle disadvantages of LDV are that it is impossible to calibrate in absolute units [28], and that it is very sensitive to artifacts from movement of the probe or underlying tissue. Furthermore, the effect of dermal configuration, epidermal thickness, and hemoglobin content of the blood is not known. Therefore, although LDV is easy to use, gives real time output, and is able to measure minute blood flow, it is difficult to perform true quantitative measurements [25].

The "micro-livedo" configuration of the upper horizontal plexus as described in the Anatomy and Physiology section above, is an important source of variation in skin blood flow measurements. The arteriolar-rich and relatively avascular zones cause a so-called *spatial heterogeneity*, i.e., the variation in LDV derived flow values from one site to another several millimeters away from the first. The aforementioned vasomotion is responsible for "temporal heterogeneity," the variation in LDV derived flow values of the same site over a period of time [3]. Although additional filtering and averaging of multiple readings may partially overcome spatial and temporal heterogeneities, it makes LDV somewhat difficult to interpret.

Skin perfusion pressure (SPP)

Predicting healing of ischemic ulcerations and amputation wounds has also been attempted by measuring the skin perfusion pressure (SPP) [7, 9]. SPP was originally defined as the external pressure needed to stop the microcirculatory washout of an intradermal depot of a radioactive tracer [10]. Simpler and faster methods of measuring the pressure of flow cessation or initiation were developed using PPG and LDV [5, 11, 18]. In a recent study, LDV assisted measurement of SPP was established as a reliable alternative to the radionuclide washout method, but PPG tracings were found to be difficult to interpret [17].

In contrast to noninvasive tests of ankle brachial indices or segmental blood pressures, SPP is not affected by intramural calcification in the media of macro vessels. This is especially important in assessing skin microcirculation in diabetic patients.

Clinical results

A perfect test would produce consistent results when repeated under the same conditions and it would reflect exactly the phenomenon that the test intended to measure. The first condition which implies complete reproducibility is almost impossible to achieve in assessing skin microcirculation, considering the various physiological functions of the skin and its spatial and temporal heterogeneities. The second condition, complete accuracy, is hampered by the complexity of both the architecture of the skin vasculature and the physical characteristics of the signals derived from the skin by the available noninvasive modalities.

It is too simplistic to expect that a single parameter could accurately stratify PAOD patients, predict lesion healing and determine amputation levels and also enhance the objective evaluation of the effect of pharmacological or other treatments.

The interpretation of test results depends on the various clinical scenarios. Prediction of healing may have totally different clinical implications than prediction of failure of healing. A test that is very good in predicting healing (high positive predictive value) may be inaccurate in the lower test range and thus be of less value in predicting failure (low negative predictive value).

Stratifying PAOD patients

The identification and stratification of patients with PAOD is important for vascular surgeons to discriminate between patients that should be considered for revascularization and those needing a more conservative approach. Noninvasive methods measuring skin microcirculation are not very helpful in evaluating the site and type (stenosis or occlusion) of arterial occlusive disease. The strength of these methods therefore is in detecting PAOD.

The diagnostic accuracy of $tcpO_2$ is dependent on the criteria for the diagnosis of symptomatic PAOD. In this respect, Scheffler and Rieger [22] collected 465 controls and 1034 symptomatic PAOD patients from the literature. For $tcpO_2$ thresholds of 40 mmHg, they found a sensitivity of 56% and a specificity of 98%. With a threshold of 50 mmHg, the figures were 72% and 86%. With the same thresholds, corresponding sensitivities/specificities for claudicants (Fontaine's stage II) were 39%/99% and 65%/93%, respectively. Therefore, only Fontaine's stage III (restpain) and IV (tissue loss), and not stage II could be distinguished from normals by means of resting $tcpO_2$. Although the poor sensitivity in claudicants has been improved by reactive hyperaemia of ergometry, $tcpO_2$ does not appear to be suitable for this stage of disease. This is in accordance with our experience, as we found $tcpO_2$ measurements helpful in stratifying patients with critical ischemia, especially in diabetic patients [6].

Confirming critical ischemia is another effort in dally practice of dealing with PAOD patients. Generally about 50% of all feet in PAOD stage III/IV show a 0 mmHg $tcpO_2$. A 10 mmHg threshold for confirming critical ischemia offers a diagnostic sensitivity of 70% and specificity of 90%.

Using LDV blood flow velocity and pulse wave amplitude with local heating and reactive hyperemia, Walden et al. [29] achieved a 96% sensitivity and specificity separating normal from ischemic limbs and a 100% accurate distinction between moderate and severely ischemic limbs. As the gold standard a combination of signs and symptoms together with ankle-brachial indices, pulse volume recordings and arteriographies was used. Although these data look promising, it is important to realize that this study concerned a limited number of subjects (50 normal, 52 moderately, and 22 severely ischemic limbs). Furthermore, two different test parameters were used and cutoff points were retrospectively determined to yield the highest possible accuracy in the sample population. The same thresholds in a different set of subjects may not prove to be so accurate. If diagnostic accuracy reaches levels this high, the validity of the gold standard to which the test results were compared must be questioned itself.

In conclusion, it appears that the initial evaluation of a patient with PAOD can be performed more reliably by clinical examination and conventional noninvasive hemodynamic techniques (ABI, ergometry and PVR) [22].

Lesion healing and selection of amputation level

Supine foot $tcpO_2$ limits from 10 to 40 mmHg have been proposed to predict healing of skin lesions [22]. In stage III/IV ischemia, postural $tcpO_2$ below 35 mmHg did not allow surgical or conservative limb salvage [22]. Unfortunately, the above mentioned flow-insensitive range of $tcpO_2$ measurements is responsible for the fact that even hypoxic supine $tcpO_2$ levels of 0 mmHg cannot rule out a successful amputation.

Scheffler and Rieger [22] also accumulated $tcpO_2$ values and clinical outcomes of 606 amputations. In 113 cases (18.6%) surgical revision at a more proximal level was required. These collated series yielded a negative predictive value (predicting failure of healing) of 70% and 50% at a 10 and 20 mmHg threshold, respectively. Relying on these $tcpO_2$ thresholds, 30% and 50% of amputations, respectively, would be performed too far proximal [22]. Alternatively, $tcpO_2$ measurement appeared an excellent predictor of lower extremity wound healing (positive predictive values of 90% and 92% at threshold of 10 and 20 mmHg, respectively). The same values were found in a recent study comparing LDV and $tcpO_2$ as predictors of wound healing in 51 amputations and 29 ulcerations [19]. Higher cutoff values produce higher positive predictive values. However, the utility of a high threshold in the clinical situation is reduced because of the corresponding poor sensitivity and negative predictive value (healing in $\pm 50\%$ of predicted failures). Thus, while this criterion may be of value in the individual patient, it is not appropriate for more general application.

Using a laser Doppler with a heated probe (45 °C) (LDHP), analyzing peak skin flow and range (peak minus minimum skin flow) during a 1-min recording, Padberg, et al. [19] achieved 100% specificity and positive predictive value for healing, but again with an unacceptable low sensitivity and negative predictive value. For predicting failures, however, a sensitivity and negative predictive value of 100% could be established using the LDHP range, while retaining a positive predictive value and accuracy of 83% and 85%, respectively.

Although PPG appeared to be very sensitive to small decreases in perfusion pressure in an experimental model [16], no clinical useful thresholds for predicting wound healing could be determined [17].

SPP using the radioisotope washout technique was found to be accurate in predicting healing of ulcerations and amputations in ischemic limbs [7, 9]. With SPP of 30 mmHg or greater, 90% of amputations healed and with SPP below 20 mmHg only 25% healed [8, 12]. Farls and Duncan [7] found that only 1 of 21 wounds with SPP below 40 mmHg healed, whereas 35 of 40 wounds with SPP above 40 mmHg healed.

Using noninvasive means of measuring the SPP to predict wound healing, LDV was found to be a valuable tool, but no clear deflection point was found using PPG [5, 17].

Evaluation of pharmacological trials

The value of $tcpO_2$ is limited because of the required heating of the skin. Vasodilatory drugs may cause a paradoxical decrease of measured $tcpO_2$ in the heated skin contrary to the non-heated skin. LDV has proved to be very useful in measuring pharmacodynamic responses to drugs [27]. PPG was also successfully used to demonstrate the action of drugs on skin microcirculation in patients with PAOD.

Conclusions

There is no "gold standard" method of measuring skin blood flow. The complex anatomy and physiology of the skin microcirculation, combined with the difficulty in fully understanding what each method measures, has led to unreliability in basing clinical decisions on measured values. Nevertheless, the three methods described in this review are far more accurate than measuring ABI and segmental pressures.

In patients with PAOD, reduced tcpO$_2$ values indicate reduced hyperemic oxygen delivery rather than real tissue hypoxia. TcpO$_2$ measurements are of no practical meaning in claudicants but in complicated PAOD. TcpO$_2$ is not useful in treatment-effect investigations because the non-heated skin microcirculation may be reflected inversely by the tcpO$_2$ signal. Very low tcpO$_2$ levels may be helpful in selecting amputation levels, predicting wound healing, and confirming critical ischemia.

PPG cannot differentiate between nutritional capillary flow and flow through deeper anastomosing vessels. It merely gives an indication of the pulsatile flow and the total blood content in the peripheral circulation. PPG is not quantitative and comparison between individuals or temporal changes within a single individual are not possible. In addition, PPG was not found to be able to measure SPP accurately. On the other hand, LDV assisted measurement of SPP may be of value if proved repeatable.

The three different methods described in this review sample different parameters and may therefore be used complementarily. The type of clinical information and its interpretation dictate the relevance of one or more investigations.

References

1. Bongard O, Bounameaux H (1993) Clinical investigation of skin microcirculation. Dermatology 186:6−11
2. Braverman IM (1989) Ultrastructure and organization of the cutaneous microvasculature in normal and pathological states. J Invest Dermatol 93:2S−9S
3. Braverman IM, Schechner JS (1991) Contour mapping of the cutaneous microvasculature by computerized laser Doppler velocimetry. J Invest Dermatol 97:1013−1018
4. Braverman IM, Yen A (1977) Ultrastructure of the human dermal microcirculation. II. The capillary loops of the dermal papillal. J Invest Dermatol 68:44−52
5. Castronuovo JJ Jr, Pabst TS, Flanigan DP, Foster LG (1987) Noninvasive determination of skin perfusion pressure using a laser Doppler. J Cardiovasc Surg 28:253−257
6. Cina C, Katsamouris A, Megerman J, Brewster DC, Strayhorn EC, Robison JG, Abbott WM (1984) Utility of transcutaneous oxygen tension measurements in peripheral arterial occlusive disease. J Vasc Surg 1:362−371
7. Farls I, Duncan H (1985) Skin perfusion pressure in the prediction of healing in diabetic patients with ulcers or gangrene of the foot. J Vasc Surg 2:536−540
8. Holstein P, Dovey H, Lassen NA (1979) Wound healing in above knee amputations in relation to skin perfusion pressure. Acta Orthop Scand 50:59−66
9. Holstein P, Lassen NA (1980) Healing of ulcers of the feet correlation with distal blood pressure measurements in occlusive arterial disease. Acta Orthop Scand 51:995−1006
10. Holstein P, Nielsen PE, Barras J-P (1979) Blood flow cessation at external pressure in the skin of normal human limbs. Microvasc Res 17:71−79
11. Holstein P, Nielsen PE, Lund P, Gyntelberg F, Poulsen HL (1980) Skin perfusion pressure on the legs measured as the external pressure required for skin reddening after blanching: a photoelectric technique compared to isotope washout. Scan J Clin Lab 40:535−543
12. Holstein P, Sager P, Lassen NA (1979) Wound healing in below knee amputations in relation to skin perfusion pressure. Acta Orthop Scand 50:49−58
13. Holzer P (1992) Peptidergic sensory neurons in the control of vascular functions: mechanisms and significance in the cutaneous and splanchnic vascular beds. Rev Physiol Biochem Pharmacol 121:49−146
14. Huch R, Huch A, Lubbers DW (1973) Transcutaneous measurement of blood pO$_2$ (TcpO$_2$)-method and application. J Perinat Med 1:183−191

15. Katsamouris A, Brewster DC, Megerman J, Cina C, Darling RC, Abbott WM (1984) Transcutaneous oxygen tension in selection of amputation level. Am J Surg 147:510–517
16. Kvernebo K, Megerman J, Hamilton G, Abbott WM (1989) Response of skin photoplethysmography, laser Doppler flowmetry and transcutaneous oxygen tensiometry to stenosis-induced reductions in limb blood flow. Eur J Vasc Surg 3:113–120
17. Maivezzi L, Castronuovo JJ Jr, Swayne LC; Cone D, Trivino JZ (1992) The correlation between three methods of skin perfusion pressure measurement; radionuclide washout, laser Doppler flow, and photoplethysmography. J Vasc Surg 15:823–829; discuss
18. Nielsen PE, Poulsen HL, Gyntelberg F (1973) Arterial blood pressure in the skin measured by a photoelectric probe and external counterpressure. Vasa 2:65–74
19. Padberg FT Jr, Back TL, Hart LC, Franco CD (1992) Comparison of heated-probe laser Doppler and transcutaneous oxygen measurements for predicitng outcome of ischemic wounds. J Cardiovasc Surg 33:715–722
20. Rithalia SV (1991) Developments in transcutaneous blood gas monitoring; a review. J Med Eng Technol 15:143–153
21. Ryan TJ (1973) Section B. Blood vessels. In: Jarrett A (ed) The physiology and pathophysiology of the skin. Volume 2. Academic press, New York, London, pp 577–805
22. Scheffler A, Rieger H (1992) Clinical information content of transcutaneous oxymetry (tcpO$_2$) in peripheral arterial occlusive disease (a review of the methodological and clinical literature with a special reference to critical limb ischaemia). Vasa 21:111–126
23. Sinclair D (1973) Section A. Nerves. In: Jarrett A (ed) The physiology and pathophysiology of the skin. Volume 2. Academic press, New York, London, pp 348–573
24. Stern MD (1975) In vivo evaluation of the microcirculation in the leg by in herent light scattering. Nature 254:56–58
25. Swain ID, Grant LF (1989) Methods of measuring skin blood flow. Phys Med Biol 34:151–175
26. Tonnesen KH (1978) Transcutaneous oxygen tension in imminent foot gangrene. Acta Anaesth Scand 68 (Suppl):107
27. Tur E (1991) Cutaneous blood flow. Laser Doppler velocimetry. Int J Dermatol 30:471–476
28. Vongsavan N, Matthews B (1993) Some aspects of the use of laser Doppler flow meters for recording tissue blood flow. Exp Physiol 78:1–14
29. Walden R, Bass A, Balaciano M, Modan M, Zulty L, Adar R (1992) Laser Doppler flowmetry in lower extremity ischemia: application and interpretation. Ann Vasc Surg 6:511–516
30. Wilkin JK (1989) Poiseuille, periodicity and perfusion: rhythmic oscillatory vasomotion in the skin. J Invest Dermatol 93:113S–118S

Authors's address:

Prof. William M. Abbott, M.D.
Massachusetts General Hospital
Dept. of Vascular Surgery
Ambulatory Care Center, Suite 458
15 Parkman Street
Boston, MA 02114
USA

Laser doppler fluxmetry in peripheral vascular disease

A. Scheffler

Abt. Innere Medizin (Chefarzt Prof. Dr. med. R. Eckhardt)
Evangelisches Krankenhaus, Köln, FRG

Introduction

Current skin microcirculatory methods differ in their spatial and temporal resolution and assess various intra- and subcutaneous vascular compartments. Laser Doppler fluxmetry (LDF) is characterized by its easy and non-invasive use and fast response to local changes of blood flow. Due to a measuring depth of about 1.5 mm the LDF signal reflects nutritional as well as functional fractions of the cutaneous circulation. The technique is suitable to record dynamic responses to provocational maneuvers as well as spontaneous fluctuations of skin blood flow. Presently, the LDF method has no practical meaning. It may be used to monitor physiological phenomena and pharmacological actions within the local cutaneous microcirculation [12, 13, 34].

Technical principles of laser Doppler fluxmetry

In 1975, Stern discovered that tissue blood flow can be read from the frequency shift of a monochromatic laser beam which is reflected at moving blood cells. For physiological erythrocyte flow velocities up to 2 mm/s the frequency shifts of a helium neon laser (633 nm) or a laser diode (780 nm) vary from 20 Hz to 8 kHz. In contrast to conventional ultrasound Doppler blood flow measurements, the theory of laser Doppler fluxmetry assumes a statistical process [40, 43]:

- Incident and reflected light are scattered randomly independent of blood content and velocity.
- Tissue hematocrit is sufficiently low to avoid multiple reflections and frequency shifts of single photons.
- Erythrocytes are distributed homogeneously and move without preferential direction.
- The average number of frequency shifts correlates linearly with the tissue hematocrit.

Assuming such a model, all blood cell velocities within a tissue specimen are assessed independently of their direction and are represented by a spectrum of Doppler frequency shifts. The demodulation of the frequency-shifted reflected light is performed automatically by the photodetector. When receiving light with two different frequencies its output signal contains a beat with a frequency proportional to the frequency difference of the two incoming signals (Doppler effect). The frequency spectrum of the photodetector signal contains these beat frequencies (velocities) within a bandwith from 20 Hz to 20 kHz. In principle, common LDF signal processors determine an arbitrarily scaled laser Doppler flux (LDF)

$$\text{laser Doppler flux} = \begin{array}{c}\text{mean}\\ \text{velocity}\\ \text{of blood cells}\end{array} \cdot \begin{array}{c}\text{tissue}\\ \text{concentration}\\ \text{of blood cells}\end{array} \quad [\text{AU}]\ .$$

It is derived by integrating the instantaneous spectral power density $P(f)$ multiplied by the corresponding frequency f

$$\mathrm{LDF} = a \cdot \int_{f_1}^{f_2} f \cdot P(f)\, df$$

over the range from f_1 to f_2. Inappropriate manufacturer or user setting of these boundaries may lead to significant measuring errors by excluding low and high erythrocyte velocities [11]. The factor a varies among the different commercial laser Doppler fluxmeters and is, for example, used to linearize the LDF signal also for high tissue hematocrits [40].

Measuring artefacts play an important practical role. They mainly result from frequency fluctuations of the laser source and movements of light conductors and the proband [40].

Methodological principles of laser Doppler fluxmetry

Measuring volume

Due to an emitted power of about 2 mW the LDF technique registers, besides the superficial capillaries, mainly the intracutaneous plexus and the thermoregulatory functional arterio-venous anastomoses. Thus, selective information about the nutritional skin circulation is not available. When orthostatic and dynamic provocational tests alter skin blood content and thereby also the measuring volume the corresponding signal changes might only partially by interpreted in terms of physiological phenomena [11, 40].

Calibration

The linear correlation of the LDF signal and the product of hematocrit times flow velocity currently used to interpret the laser Doppler output was determined by means of an in-vitro flow chamber [31]. These results, however, could not be reproduced in a recent study where flux values vaired extremely with the hematocrit [11].

The LDF method was compared in animals as well as in humans with several other techniques for measuring tissue blood flow. Despite good intraindividual qualitative correlations a large quantitative intra- as well as interindividual scatter was observed, making a general flow calibration of the LDF signal impossible [11, 17, 36, 41, 42]. To ensure long-term stability and to minimize variations between different equipment an adjustment of the signal processor by means of standardized latex particle suspensions has been recommended [40].

Biological zero

When a LDF probe is directed against a light-reflecting stationary non-biological material the processor outputs the electronical zero value. However, in biological tissues during a circulatory arrest or post mortem and even in meat slices usually an non-zero flux value is obtained referred to as the "biological zero" (BZ). In vascular patients the BZ value often represents the major portion of the total LDF value. The BZ increases with rising tissue temperatures and may result from Brown's corpuscular movements, maintained vasomotion, and blood cell sedimentation. In practice, the BZ should always be determined by means of a short arterial occlusion and subtracted from all subsequent LDF readings [6, 40, 52].

Biological variability and reproducibility

At rest LDF values exhibit a large spatial and temporal fluctuation. In consequence, individual LDF measurements have a poor reproducibility [9, 18, 35, 45, 47].

Results in patients with peripheral arterial occlusive disease (PAOD)

Measurements at rest

Several groups have demonstrated that an impaired resting skin perfusion cannot be observed by means of laser Doppler fluxmetry in PAOD patients proximal to the toes. Occasionally, even increased basal fluxes were found in claudicants. Significantly reduced LDF values were only derived at the toes in limb-threatening critical ischemia [5, 10, 12, 18, 23, 32, 34, 44, 51, 53].

Provocational tests

Pathological alterations of skin microcirculation in PAOD patients are best assessed by means of provocational maneuvers which test either physiological meachanisms of blood flow regulation (positional changes, venous occlusion, local cooling) or the functional flow reserve (postocclusive reactive hyperemia, local heating).

– *Heating of the LDF probe*
  Heating the LDF probe to temperatures above 40 °C induces a local hyperemia. As compared to healthy controls PAOD patients exhibit a smaller flux increase due to their reduced flow reserve [9, 35, 53].

– *Postocclusive reactive hyperemia*
  A reactive hyperemia can be provoked by means of a temporary arterial cuff occlusion at the thigh, calf, or toe levels. The LDF signal is recorded continuously at rest and during the period of hyperemia. From these tracings parameters like the peak flux, the flux reappearance time, the half-time of flux recovery, the flux recovery time, the time-to-peak flux, the half-time of hyperemia, or the time of hyperemia can be derived.
  A good discrimination between normals and PAOD patients was obtained after a 3 min circulatory arrest with the cuff positioned at the thigh when the initial

phase of the hyperemic reaction during cuff deflation and peak flux was considered. In healthy persons the time to peak flux takes about $10-25$ s. Thereby, the peak flux amounts to $3-10$ times that of the resting flux. In claudicants the peak flux is delayed to $40-150$ s and reaches only $1.5-3$ times of the basal value. In critical limb ischemia frequently a reactive hyperemia cannot be induced at distal parts of the leg [5, 9, 10, 18, 21, 22, 25, 26, 32, 35, 51].

— *Positional changes*
Increasuing the arteriolar or venolar transmural pressure leads to a physiological vasoconstriction. Accordingly, leg dependency or a venous occlusion are accompanied by a corresponding drop of the LDF signal. In healthy controls LDF values fall to $25-50\%$ of the horizontal readings when the leg is lowered. In claudicants this LDF reaction is reduced on average to $0-25\%$. Furthermore, signal increases can be observed from time to time which indicate an abolished local flow control. The latter phenomenon predominates in critical limb ischemia [3, 9, 12, 26, 34, 48, 49, 51].

Analysis of temporal LDF patterns

The continuously recorded LDF signal includes integrated information on the local temporal behavior of various microcirculatory mechanisms of flow control. Prony spectral analysis, discrete Fourier transformation, and digital filtering have been introduced to differentiate these processes inside the frequency domain. However, the clinical and biological impact of these approaches still remains to be clarified. Besides such numerical procedures, descriptive classifications of LDF tracings according to predominating signal patterns and frequencies have been described [9, 14, 15, 28, 37−39].

In vascular patients, temporal fluctuations of the LDF skin perfusion seem to vary with hemodynamic compensation and clinical staging. The amplitude of pulse synchronous LDF oscillations is attenuated with increasing severity of PAOD until it is completely erased in critical ischemia. Aperiodical or periodical flux oscillations of high amplitude and low frequency (<10 min^{-1}) predominate in cases with sufficient skin circulation. In critical ischemia, however, usually small LDF fluctuations with high frequency ($15-20$ min^{-1}) or even missing flux motions are observed. Such "small" or "high frequency" waves obviously indicate a passive flux behavior governed by respiratory fluctuations of venous pressures typical for ischemic skin areas. They disappear after a successful revascularization [13−15, 18, 29, 38, 39].

Measurement of acral perfusion pressures

— *Digital arterial pressures*
A LDF sensor can be applied to detect the reoccurrence of blood flow after a suprasystolic arterial cuff occlusion at various sites of a limb including the toes. Systolic arterial pressures measured by the LDF technique correlated well with values obtained by means of the conventional strain-gauge method. LDF sensors are applicable even in toes with difficult anatomic conditions [1, 2, 20].

138

– Skin perfusion pressures
The skin perfusion pressure is usually defined by an externally applied pressure
which causes a flow stop in the underlying skin area. The local perfusion can be
recorded by a LDF probe incorporated into a pressure cuff. Skin perfusion
pressures obtained by means of LDF cuff sensors correlated well with those measured by conventional isotope clearance techniques [8, 27, 32, 44].

Critical limb ischemia and prediction of wound healing

Patients with critical limb ischemia constitute the target group for practical applications of skin microcirulatory measurements. So far, reports available on the prediction of ischemic skin lesions by means of LDF readings are rather contradictory.
LDF measurement were obtained at rest and with probes heated to 44 °C. Also am-
plitudes of LDF oscillations were considered. Pilot studies found a close correlation
with the tcpO$_2$ technique. However, presently the clinical meaning of the LDF method is still rather questionable [12, 16, 19, 33, 34].

Evaluation of therapeutical effects

LDF recordings can be used to monitor direct pharmacological effects on the skin
microcirculation. In general, relative signal changes at acral skin areas are evaluated
[7, 12, 24, 34]. The method may also be applied to demonstrate a sympatholytic
vasodilatation due to an epidural analgesia or spinal cord stimulation [4, 30, 46, 50].

References

1. Andersson S, Linderholm H, Rinnström O, Burlin L (1986) A laser Doppler technique for measuring distal blood pressure: a comparison with conventional strain-gauge technique. Clin
   Physiol 6:329–335
2. Beinder E, Hoffmann U, Franzeck UK, Huch A, Huch R, Bollinger A (1992) Laser Doppler
   technique for the measurement of digital and segmental systolic blood pressure. Vasa 21:15–21
3. Belcaro G, Vasdekis S, Rulo A, Nicolaides AN (1989) Evaluation of skin blood flow and
   venoarteriolar response in patients with diabetes and peripheral vascular disease by laser Doppler flowmetry. Angiology 40:953–957
4. Bengtsson M (1984) Changes in skin blood flow and temperature during spinal analgesia evaluated by laser Doppler flowmetry and infrared thermography. Acta Anaesthesiol Scand
   28:625–630
5. Bongard O, Fagrell B (1990) Discrepancies between total and nutritional skin microcirculation
   in patients peripheral arterial occlusive disease (PAOD). Vasa 19:105–111
6. Caspary L, Creutzig A, Alexander K (1988) Biological zero in laser Doppler fluxmetry. Int J
   Microcirc: Clin Exp 7:367–371
7. Caspary L, Creutzig A, Alexander K (1991) Intravenous infusion of iloprost in arterial occlusive disease: dose-dependent effects on skin microcirculation. Eur J Clin Pharmacol
   41:131–136
8. Castronouvo JJ, Pabst TS, Flanigan DP, Foster LG (1987) Noninvasive determination of skin
   perfusion pressure using a laser Doppler. J Cardiovasc Surg 28:253–257
9. Creutzig A, Caspary L, Hertel RF, Alexander K (1987) Temperature-dependent laser Doppler
   fluxmetry in healthy and patients with peripheral arterial occlusive disease. Int J Microcirc:
   Clin Exp 6:381–390

10. del Guercio R, Leonardo G, Arpaia MR (1986) Evaluation of postischemic hyperemia on the skin using laser Doppler velocimetry: Study on patients with claudicatio intermittens. Microvasc Res 32:289–299

11. Driessen G, Rütten W, Inhoffen W, Scheidt H, Heidtmann H (1990) Is the laser Doppler flow signal a measure of microcirculatory cell flux? Int J Microcirc: Clin Exp 9:141–161

12. Fagrell B (1990) Peripheral vascular diseases. In: Shepherd AP, Öberg PA (eds) Laser-Doppler blood flowmetry. Kluwer Academic Publishers, Boston Dordrecht London, pp 201–213

13. Hoffmann U, Franzeck UK, Bollinger A (1992) Laser-Doppler-Technik bei Krankheiten der peripheren Gefäße. Dtsch Med Wschr 117:1889–1897

14. Hoffmann U, Schneider E, Bollinger A (1990) Flow motion waves with high and low frequency in severe ischaemia before and after percutaneous transluminal angioplasty. Cardiovasc Res 24:711–718

15. Hoffmann U, Yanar A, Franzeck UK, Edwards JM, Bollinger A (1990) The frequency histogram – A new method for the evaluation of laser Doppler flux motion. Microvasc Res 40:293–301

16. Holloway GA, Burgess EM (1983) Preliminary experience with laser Doppler velocimetry for the determination of amputation levels. Prosthet Orthot Inter 7:63–66

17. Holloway GA, Watkins DW (1977) Laser Doppler measurement of cutaneous blood flow. J Invest Dermatol 69:306–309

18. Karanfilian RG, Lynch TG, Lee BC, Long JB, Hobson RW (1984) The assessment of skin blood flow in peripheral vascular disease by laser Doppler velocimetry. Am Surg 50:641–644

19. Karanfilian RG, Lynch TG, Zirul VT, Padberg FT, Jamil Z, Hobson RW (1986) The value of laser Doppler velocimetry and transcutaneous oxygen tension determination in predicting healing of ischemic forefoot ulcerations and amputations in diabetic and nondiabetic patients. J Vasc Surg 4:511–516

20. Kristensen JK, Engelhardt M, Nielsen T (1983) Laser-Doppler measurement of digital blood flow regulation in normals and in patients with Raynaud's phenomenon. Acta Derm Venereol (Stockh) 63:43–47

21. Kvernebo K, Slagsvold CE, Gjolberg T (1988) Laser Doppler flux reappearence time (FRT) in patients with lower limb atherosclerosis and healthy controls. Eur J Vasc Surg 2:171–176

22. Kvernebo K, Slagsvold CE, Stranden E (1989) Laser Doppler flowmetry in evaluation of skin post-ischaemic reactive hyperaemia. J Cardiovasc Surg 30:70–75

23. Kvernebo K, Slagsvold CE, Stranden E, Kroese A, Larsen S (1988) Laser Doppler flowmetry in evaluation of lower limb resting skin circulation – A study in healthy controls and atherosclerotic patients. Scand J Clin Lab Invest 48:621–626

24. Leonardo G, Arpaia MR, del Guercio R (1986) Evaluation of the effects of vasoactive drugs on cutaneous microcirculation by laser Doppler velocimetry. Angiology 37:12–19

25. Leonardo G, Arpaia MR, del Guercio R (1987) A new method for the quantitative assessment of arterial insufficiency of the limbs: Cutaneous postischemic hyperemia test by laser Doppler. Angiology 38:378–385

26. Lerche A, Paaske WP (1986) Laser Doppler examination of peripheral microvascular reactivity. Surg Gynecol Obstet 163:410–414

27. Malvezzi L, Castronuovo JJ Jr, Swayne LC, Cone D, Trivino JZ (1992) The correlation between three methods of skin perfusion measurement: radionuclide washout, laser Doppler flow, and plethysmography. J Vasc Surg 15:823–829

28. Meyer JU, Burkhard PM, Secomb TW, Intaglietta M (1989) The Prony spectral line estimation (PSLE) method for the analysis of vascular oscillations. IEEE Trans Biomed Eng 36:968–971

29. Moneta GL, Schneider E, Jäger K, Brülisauer M, Thüring-Vollenweider U, Bollinger A (1988) Laser Doppler flux and vasomotion in patients before and after transluminal angioplasty for limb salvage. Vasa 17:26–31

30. Naver H, Augustinsson LE, Elam M (1992) The vasodilating effect of spinal dorsal column stimulation is mediated by sympathetic nerves. Clin Auton Res 2:41–45

31. Nilsson GE, Tenland T, Öberg PA (1980) Evaluation of a laser Doppler flowmeter for measurement of tissue blood flow. IEEE Trans Biomed Eng 27:597–604

32. Pabst TS, Castronouvo JJ, Jackson SD, Schuler JJ, Flanigan DP (1985) Evaluation of the ischemic limb by pressure and flow measurements of the skin microcirculation as determined by laser Doppler velocimetry. Curr Surg 42:29–31

33. Padberg FT Jr, Back TL, Hart LC, Franco CD (1992) Comparison of heated-probe laser Doppler and transcutaneous oxygen measurements for predicting outcome of ischemic wounds. J Cardiovasc Surg 33:715–722
34. Ranft J (1988) Stellenwert der Laser-Doppler-Untersuchung bei Patienten mit arterieller Verschlußkrankheit. Herz 13:382–391
35. Ranft J, Heidrich H, Peters A, Trampisch H (1986) Laser-Doppler examinations in persons with healty vasculature and in patients with peripheral arterial occlusive disease. Angiology 37:818–827
36. Saumet JL, Dittmar A, Leftheriotis G (1986) Non-invasive measurement of skin blood flow: comparison between plethysmography, laser-Doppler-flowmeter and heat thermal clearance method. Int J Microcirc: Clin Exp 5:73–83
37. Scheffler A, Rieger H (1990) A microcomputer system for evaluation of laser Doppler blood flux measurements. In J Microcirc: Clin Exp 9:357–368
38. Scheffler A, Rieger H (1992) Spontaneous oscillations of laser Doppler skin blood flux in peripheral arterial occlusive disease. Int J Microcirc: Clin Exp 11:249–261
39. Seifert H, Jäger K, Bollinger A (1988) Analysis of flow motion by the laser Dopplert technique in patients with peripheral arterial occlusive disease. Int J Microcirc: Clin Exp 7:223–236
40. Shepherd AP, Öberg PA (eds) (1990) Laser-Doppler blood flowmetry. Kluwer Academic Publishers, Boston Dordrecht London
41. Shepherd AP, Riedel GL, Kiel JW, Haumschild DJ, Maxwell LC (1987) Evaluation of an infrared laser Doppler blood flowmeter. Am J Physiol 252:G832–G839
42. Smits GJ, Roman RJ, Lombard JH (1986) Evaluation of laser-Doppler flowmetry as a measure of tissue blood flow. J Appl Physiol 61:666–672
43. Stern MD (1975) In vivo evaluation of microcirculation by coherent light scattering. Nature 254:56–58
44. Svensson H, Bornmyr S, Svedman P (1990) Skin perfusion pressure assessed by measuring the external pressure required to stop blood cell flux. Angiology 41:169–174
45. Tenland T, Salerud EG, Nilsson GE, Öberg PA (1983) Spatial and temporal variations in human skin blood flow. Int J Microcirc: Clin Exp 2:81–90
46. Thomson MB, Lassvik V, Bengtsson M (1988) Changes in skin perfusion after sympathetic block with Guanethidine – Laser Doppler fluxmetry in human volunteers. Int J Microcirc: Clin Exp 7:123–130
47. Tur E, Tur M, Maibach HI, Guy RH (1983) Basal perfusion of the cutaneous microcirulation: Measurements as a function of anatomic position. J Invest Dermatol 81:442–446
48. Ubbink D, Jacobs M, Slaaf D, Tangelder G, Reneman R (1992) Microvascular reactivity differences between two legs of patients with unilateral lower limb ischaemia. Eur J Vasc Surg 6:269–275
49. Ubbink D, Kitslaar P, Tordoir J, Tangelder G, Reneman R, Jacobs M (1992) The relevance of posturally induced microvascular constriction after revascularisation in patients with chronic leg ischaemia. Eur J Vasc Surg 6:525–532
50. Valley MA, Bourke DL, Hamill MP, Raja SN (1993) Time course of sympathetic blockade during epidural anesthesia: laser Doppler flowmetry studies of regional skin perfusion. Anesth Analg 76:289–294
51. Wahlberg E, Jörneskog G, Olofsson P, Swedenborg J, Fagrell B (1990) The influence of reactive hyperemia and leg dependency on skin microcirculation in patients with peripheral arterial occlusive disease (PAOD), with and without diabetes. Vasa 19:301–306
52. Wahlberg E, Olofsson P, Swedenborg J, Fagrell B (1992) Effects of local hyperemia and edema on the biological zero in laser Doppler fluxmetry (LD). Int J Microcirc: Clin Exp 11:157–165
53. Winsor T, Haumschild DJ, Winsor D, Mikail A (1989) Influence of local and environmental temperatures on cutaneous circulation with use of laser Doppler flowmetry. Angiology 40:421–428

Authors' address:

PD Dr. med. Andreas Scheffler
Abt. Innere Medizin
Evangelisches Krankenhaus, Weyertal 76
D-50931 Köln, FRG

Clinical evaluations

Transcutaneous oxygen tension in patients with critical limb ischemia treated by spinal cord stimulation

L. Claeys, K. Ktenidis, S. Horsch

Academic Teaching Hospital Cologne-Porz, FRG

Introduction

In patients with PAOD, critical blood supply of muscle tissue and skin causes pain at rest and acral skin necrosis or gangrene. Pain at rest is usually localized in the forefoot. It is a severe pain, often continuous and typically worsening at night.

Vascular reconstruction is the treatment of choice for patients with severe PAOD, Fontaine Stages III and IV [13] and it has increased foot salvage. Despite this progress the number of non-reconstructable patients still remains high [16]. This leaves medical pain treatment and amputation as the only alternatives available.

The ideal treatment in these stages should allow the patient to retain his limb with no or tolerable pain and to regain a satisfactory level of independence.

Spinal cord stimulation was first introduced into clinical practice for the treatment of intractable pain [22, 25]. Cook (1973) noticed an improvement in lower limb blood flow in a group of patients who were being treated with SCS for pain related to multiple sclerosis [7, 8]. He investigated the use of SCS as a method of pain control for severe ischemic pain. Other early clinical reports on ESCS reported pain relief and healing of ischemic ulcers in endstage vascular patients, suggesting that ESCS improves nutritional blood flow [2, 3, 5, 6, 10, 11, 14, 17]. Jacobs (1988) using capillary microscopy, found that during ESCS the number of skin capillaries perfused and skin capillary red blood cell velocity were significantly increased. These findings could explain the observed clinical improvement and ulcer healing in patients with PAOD treated with ESCS [19].

Non-invasive diagnostic techniques have been used to attempt the effect of ESCS on peripheral blood flow but were not sensitive enough [9].

Transcutaneous oximetry is an indirect non-invasive method for the evaluation of skin perfusion. Although, several factors influence $TcPO_2$, it is gaining acceptance as a simple and effective means of evaluating the cutaneous circulation [12, 18, 20]. This paper reports our clinical experience and our long-term observations of $TcPO_2$ in patients with non-reconstructable PAOD of the lower limbs treated with ESCS.

Patients and methods

From January 1986 to December 1991, 177 patients with non-reconstructable PAOD of the lower limbs were treated by ESCS. PAOD was attributed to arteriosclerosis in all patients, 36 of them had also diabetic vascular disease. The patients, 68 women and 109 men, ranged in age from 45 to 83 years with a mean of 67.3 years. Clinical status was classified as stage III in 114 patients and as stage IV in 63 patients. The diagnosis was confirmed by ankle/brachial blood pressure index (ABI) less than

0.40, by angiographic findings and by $TcPO_2$ measured on the dorsum of the foot. The intensity of the symptoms was rated by the patient as severe in all cases. The duration of the medical history ranged from 3.6 months to more than 5 years. Angiograms, either intraarterial or intraoperative, showed occluded cruval vessels unsuitable for a bypass procedure or angioplasty. Prior to the implantation all patients had received conservative treatment, 159 had undergone one or more failed bypass procedures on the involved leg, and 23 had a lumbar sympathectomy. All patients had ischemic rest pain for at least 2 weeks. Patients with significant heart failure, pulmonary or renal insufficiency, unstable angina, hypertension (SBP > 180 mmHg) were excluded. No platelet-inhibiting drugs, anticoagulants, fibrinolytic or vasoactive drugs were given.

In order to benefit from the stimulation therapy the patient must be able to understand the principles of this therapy: the stimulation will replace the pain with paresthesia and the patient must be willing to accept these paresthesia. The implantation of the ESCS system was only considered after this strict patient selection and informed consent. The process of selection requires the following steps: the patients must undergo a careful vascular evaluation, the stimulation must be used as a last resort, conservative and surgical therapies must have been attempted and failed, and professional equipment and experience for implantation and follow-up must be available (Table 1). The follow-up examinations were performed before implantation, 1 and 2 weeks postoperatively and at 3-month intervals after implantation and included analysis of pain relief, measurement of the ankle pressure and transcutaneous oxygen tension with calculation of respectively the ankle/brachial index and the regional perfusion index.

The parameters considered in our evaluation of pain relief were based upon the intake of analgesic drugs and patient self-evaluation. Systolic arterial ankle pressure was measured by ultrasonic Doppler sonography in the posterior and anterior tibial arteries and expressed in mmHg. The ankle/brachial blood pressure index (ABI), expressed as a percentage, was determined by dividing the systolic ankle pressure by the systolic brachial artery pressure.

Transcutaneous oximetry was chosen to assess the microvascular status of the skin.

The oximeter utilizes a Clark-type oxygen-sensing electrode that attaches to the skin. The heating element of the electrode is warmed to 45 °C. This minimizes local vasomotor tone and causes a maximal vasodilation and capillary opening. Capillary blood flow and, indirectly, the transcutaneous oxygen pressure is determined by:

Table 1. Patient selection

- Chronic severe ischemic rest pain
- Endstage PAOD:
    - ABI <0.4 or toe pressure <30 mmHg
    - non-reconstructable
    - no suitable vessels
    - contraindications for general anesthesia
    - failed bypass procedure (patient refuses bypass surgery)
- Ulcers/dry gangrene <3.0 cm² in diameter
- Patient cooperative and informed consent
- Life expectancy >6 months
- Pain relief during trial stimulation

capillary perfusion pressure, capillary patency, blood viscosity, arterio-venous shunting, and other factors.

The TcPO$_2$ measurements were performed with the patient resting in the supine position. The electrodes were attached on the dorsum of both feet. Measurement of the chest TcPO$_2$ was performed in order to record reference value. The ratio between foot and chest TcPO$_2$ was referred to as the Regional Perfusion Index (RPI) and can be interpreted in a manner analogous to the ankle/brachial blood pressure index (ABI).

Surgical technique

The treatment is performed by placing a quadripolar lead in the epidural space by a percutaneous lumbar puncture between L3 and L4 (PISCES – Quad 3487A Medtronic Inc.). The lead is advanced under radioscopic control to the level of Th 11 – 12. Midline placement is preferable (Fig. 1). Connecting a portable stimulator to the lead allows intraoperative test stimulation producing comfortable paresthesias in the painful foot or limb.

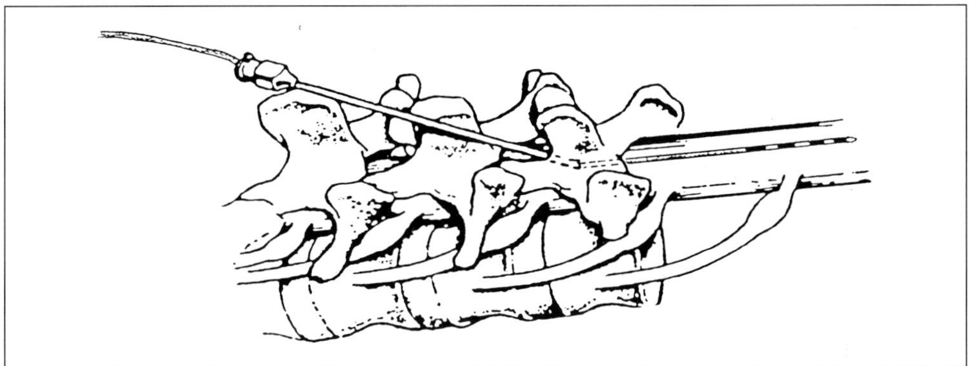

Fig. 1. The Tuohy needle is inserted through the interluminar ligament to enter the epidural space. A quadripolar electrode is placed for bipolar stimulation. The midline of the spinal cord may be displaced from the apparent anatomical midline, the surgeon must follow patient's report of the location of the paresthesias

During a trial period of 1 week the clinical effects are tested. If the patient has enjoyed significant pain relief, an implantable pulse generator (ITREL II IPG, Medtronic Inc.) is placed in a subcutaneous pocket of the abdomen. The usual initial settings are a pulse amplitude between 1.0 – 2.5 V, a frequency between 70 – 120 pps and a pulse width of 180 – 450 ms. Stimulation can be given continuously or intermittently. During follow-up the parameters can be reset with the help of a special computer.

Statistical analysis

The TcPO$_2$ data are presented as mean values and standard deviations. Paired t-tests were performed with values of $p < 0.05$ considered significant.

Table 2. Clinical results of ESCS therapy

	N	mean days usage	mean % pain relief	No amputations minor/major
Stage III		n = 114		
S:	93	38.6 m	>75%	0/0
PS:	9	6.8 m	50 – 70%	2/ – 1 AKA – 6 BKA
F:	12	2.1 m	<50%	0/ – 2 AKA – 10 BKA
Stage IV		n = 63		
S:	17	32.9 m	>75%	8/0
PS:	19	6.3 m	50 – 70%	9/ – 5 AKA – 5 BKA
F:	27	1.7 m	<50%	0/ – 17 AKA – 10 BKA

S: success; PS: partial success; F: failure
AKA: above-knee amputation
BKA: below-knee amputation

Results

The results are summarized in Table 2. Twenty-one patients died during the follow-up period, 13 due to cardiac and/or pulmonary insufficiency, one patient died from a septic shock due to a stump infection after amputation, and four from a cerebrovascular accident.

There was no method-related mortality.

We defined three types of outcome:

1) success defined as pain relief of more than 75% and avoiding an amputation;
2) partial success defined as temporary benefit with pain relief between 50 and 70% but with progression of the disease resulting in amputation after a period of success;
3) failure defined as very little pain relief resulting in limb amputation within the first 6 months and technical problems resulting in device removal.

77.9% of the patients (102 stage III and 36 stage IV) obtained complete or very good pain relief. These positive results post implant dropped slowly in 28 patients. This can be due to a loss of effectiveness of the ESCS in controlling the ischemic pain. On the other hand PAOD is a progressive disease that worsens over time. These patients occasionally needed non-narcotic analgesics.

Despite a good initial clinical effect ESCS was not able to control the ischemic pain in 21 stage III and in 46 stage IV patients. These patients underwent an amputation. An above-the-knee amputation was necessary in three stage III and in 22 stage IV patients and a below-the-knee amputation in 16 stage III and in 15 stage IV

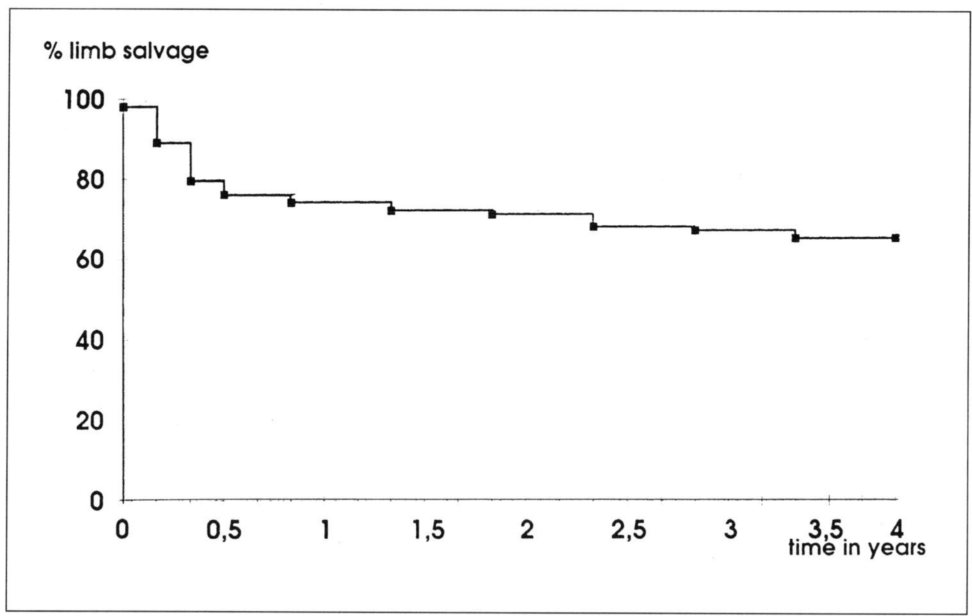

Fig. 2. Cumulative limb salvage after ESCS (Cutler-Ederer-Method)

patients. Eleven patients underwent a minor amputation, preserving a functional extremity. The limb survival rate showed a 69% 4-year survival (Fig. 2).

$TcPO_2$ foot values in the non-amputated stage III patients increased from 24.2 ± 5.5 mmHg to 48.1 ± 6.4 mmHg ($p > 0.02$) and the RPI from 0.52 to 0.91. In the non-amputated stage IV patients, $TcPO_2$ foot values showed an average improvement from a mean of 16.4 ± 6.2 mmHg to 38.2 ± 7.1 mmHg ($p < 0.03$), RPI increased from 0.33 to 0.74 (Fig. 3). No significant changes were observed in the ABI. Seven patients were lost to follow-up. No difference was found in subjective findings between patients with and without diabetes nor between patients with and without previous sympathectomy.

Technical problems occurred in 42 patients (23.7%). Lead dislocation (30 patients) and break (12 patients) were recognized by a change or a loss of the stimulation-produced paresthesias. Lead break occurred in 12 patients. After repositioning of the electrode in 10 patients the system functioned properly again.

Lead replacement was impossible in the two other cases, possibly due to the formation of fibrous tissue around the electrode. Electrode dislocation usually occurred in the first 2 months after implantation. In 22 patients with lead dislocation, replacement was necessary and posed no special difficulties. In the other eight patients comfortable paresthesias could be obtained after reprogramming. Seven patients developed an infection of the system that required removal of the device. In three patients skin necrosis occurred over the generator, in two of these cases an immediate reimplantation was possible, the other patient developed an infection of the generator pocket. Two liquor fistula complicated the procedure.

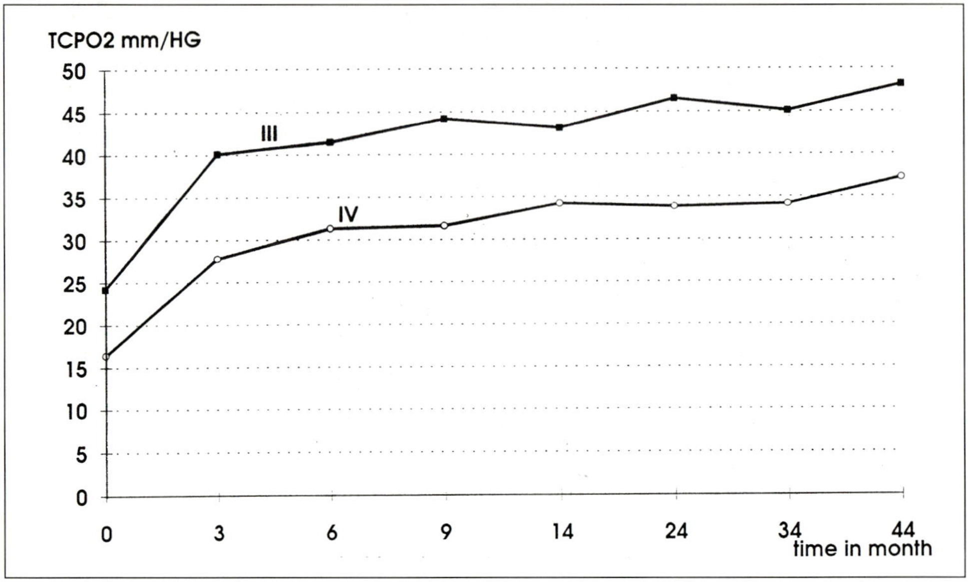

Fig. 3. Physiologic changes of TCPO2 under epidural spinal cord stimulation in stage III and IV patients with limb salvage

Discussion

The most important symptom in patients with severe PAOD is ischemic pain at rest that makes a normal life impossible. Amputation is often the only alternative for pain relief when vascular reconstruction is impossible. Since 1967, ESCS has become an accepted technique for the management of chronic pain. This has led to the use of ESCS to treat chronic ischemic pain [1, 24].

Several published reports confirmed pain relief under ESCS, suggesting an improvement of the nutritional blood flow [15, 21]. The exact mechanisms underlying the effect of ESCS on pain and peripheral blood flow remain uncertain. The neurophysiology is based on the Gate Control Theory of Pain postulated by Melzack and Wall in 1965 [26]. This theory of segmental pain inhibition suggests that the stimulation of large afferent nerve fibers in the dorsal columns of the spinal cord prevents the transmission of pain information from smaller diameter pain fibers. Pain relief may be assisted by improvement of the microcirculation due to a release of the reflex sympathetically mediated vasoconstriction that is known to occur in response to pain.

There is evidence that electrical stimulation might act by releasing endorphins and neuronal messengers like substance P [24].

We have studied the effects of ESCS in 177 patients with clinical and angiographic evidence of non-reconstructable PAOD. All patients had severe symptoms and had either failed to respond to conventional surgical and medical treatment or were unsuitable for such treatment. 77.9% of our patients immediately noted a good pain relief; this relief was most effective in stage III. TcPO$_2$ as a non-invasive method was

150

chosen as an objective assessment of the microcirculation [23]. These values showed an overall increase following the stimulation. After ESCS, $TcPO_2$ at the dorsum of the foot increased significantly. This can be interpreted as an increase in skin blood flow and explains the clinical improvement. It is unlikely that the increase in skin perfusion is caused by an improved arterial inflow since the ABI did not change significantly. In the 56 patients who went on to major amputation, $TcPO_2$ did not increase immediately. In the responder stage III patients the $TcPO_2$ rose an average of 70.5% and in the responder stage IV patients of 107%. On the basis of our experience, $TcPO_2$ measurements could be useful for predicting the efficacy of ESCS [27].

An increase of the $TcPO_2$ of at least 20 mmHg can be applied predictively to divide the patients into responders and non-responders. The best clinical results were achieved in the patients with significant $TcPO_2$ increase and in the patients with rest pain. Our attempts to demonstrate an objective correlation between the clinical effects and the physiologic changes in the microcirculation under SCS are encouraging.

We conclude that ESCS is promising in patients with severe PAOD when previous therapies have failed and arterial reconstruction is impossible. The main effect is the relief of ischemic pain. To evaluate the therapeutic effect of ESCS vis a vis limb salvage a prospective randomized study is necessary.

Summary

Epidural spinal cord stimulation (ESCS) has been suggested to improve the microcirculatory blood flow and to reduce amputation rate.

We studied the efficacy of ESCS in 177 patients with peripheral arterial occlusive disease. In all cases medical or surgical therapy had failed or vascular reconstruction was impossible. Clinical status was classified as Fontaine Stage III, chronic ischemic rest pain, in 114 patients, and as Fontaine Stage IV, rest pain with ulcers or dry gangrene, in 63 patients. PAOD was due to arteriosclerosis, 36 patients had diabetic vascular disease. After a mean follow-up period of 35.6 months, significant pain relief ($>75\%$) was obtained in the patients with limb survival. Fifty-eight patients underwent a major amputation. The limb survival rate showed a 69% 4-year survival. The systolic ankle/brachial blood pressure index was used as parameter of the macrocirculation. As parameter of the microcirculation, $TcPO_2$ was assessed on the dorsum of the foot and the regional perfusion index was calculated. Clinical improvement was confirmed by the increase in $TcPO_2$ ($p<0.02$) from 24.2 to 48.1 mmHg in the non-amputated stage III patients and from 16.4 to 37.2 mmHg in the non-amputated stage IV patients ($p<0.03$). We conclude that in patients with severe non-reconstructable PAOD of the lower limbs, ESCS improves skin blood flow and shows good pain relief, making patients life more comfortable.

References

1. Augustinsson LE, Holm J, Carlsson CA, Jivegard L (1985) Epidural electrical stimulation in severe ischaemia. Evidence of pain relief, increased blood flow and a possible limb-saving effect. Ann Surg 202:104–111
2. Augustinsson LE (1987) Epidural spinal electrical stimulation in peripheral vascular disease. Pace 10:205–206
3. Bracale GC, Selvetella L, Mirabile F (1989) Our experience with spinal cord stimulation in peripheral vascular disease. Pace 12:695–697

4. Brodin E, Linderoth B, Gazelius B, Ungestedt U (1987) In vivo release of substance P in cat dorsal horn studied with microdialysis. Neuroscience Letters, Elsevier Scientific Publishers Ireland Ltd 76:357–362

5. Broggi G, Servello D, Franzini A (1987) Spinal cord stimulation for treatment of peripheral vascular disease. Appl Neurophysiol 50:439–441

6. Broseta I, Barbara I, De Vera IA (1986) Spinal cord stimulation in peripheral arterial disease. J Neurosurgery 64:71–80

7. Cook AW, Oygar A, Baggenstos P, Pacheto S, Kleniga E (1976) Vascular disease of the extremities: electrical stimulation of the spinal cord and the posterior roots. NY State J Med 76:366–368

8. Cook AW (1980) Electrical stimulation in multiple sclerosis. Med Biol Eng Comput 18:48–56

9. Dilley RB, Fronek A (1987) Quantitative velocity measurements in arterial disease of the lower extremity. In: Bernstein EF (ed) Noninvasive Diagnostic Techniques in Vascular Disease. St. Louis, The CV Mosby Company 294–303

10. Dooley D, Kasprak M (1976) Modification of blood flow to the extremities by electrical stimulation of the nervous system. South Med J 69:1309–1311

11. Fiume D (1983) Spinal cord stimulation in peripheral vascular pain. Appl Neurophysiol 46:290–294

12. Franzeck UK, Talke P, Bernstein EF et al. (1982) Transcutaneous PO_2 measurements in health and peripheral arterial occlusive disease. Surgery 91:156–163

13. Friedman SG, Kerner BA, Friedman MS, Moccio CG (1989) Limb salvage in elderly patients. Is aggressive surgical therapy warranted? J Cardiovasc Surg 30:848–851

14. Galley D, Elharrar C, Scheffer J et al. (1989) Neurostimulation et pathologie vasculaire: intéret thérapeutique a propos de 49 patients. Coeur 20:35–44

15. Galley D, Elharrar C, Scheffer J, Jeangeorges B, Serena G (1989) Neurostimulation et pathologie vasculaire: intéret thérapeutique a propos de 49 patients. Coeur 20:35–44

16. Gregg RO (1985) Bypass or amputation. Concommitant review of bypass arterial grafting and major amputations. Am J Surg 149:397–402

17. Groth KE (1985) Spinal cord stimulation for the treatment of peripheral vascular disease. European multicenter study. In: Fields H (ed) Advances in pain research and therapy. Raven Press New York, pp 861–870

18. Hauser CL, Shoemaker WC (1983) Use of transcutaneous PO_2 regional perfusion index to quantify tissue perfusion in peripheral vascular disease. Ann Surg 197:337–343

19. Jacobs MHJM, Jörning PJG, Beckers RCY, Ubbink DT et al. (1990) Foot salvage and improvement of microvascular blood flow as a result of epidural spinal cord electrical stimulation. J Vasc Surg 12:354–360

20. Jasczak P, Poulsen J (1983) Estimation of blood flow in transcutaneous PO_2 measurements. Acta Anaesthesiol Scand 27:174

21. Jivegard L, Augustinsson LE, Carlsson CA, Holm J (1987) Longterm results by epidural spinal electrical stimulation (ESES) in patients with inoperable severe lower limb ischemia. Eur J Vasc Surg 1:345–349

22. Long DM (1977) Electrical stimulation for the control of pain. Arch Surg 122:884–888

23. Matsen F, Wyss C, Pedgena L et al. (1980) Transcutaneous oxygen tension measurements in peripheral vascular disease. Surg Gynecol Obstet 150:525–528

24. Meglio M, Cioni B (1982) Personal experience with spinal cord stimulation in chronic pain management. Appl Neurophysiol 45:195

25. Meglio M, Cioni B, Rossi GF (1989) Spinal cord stimulation in management of chronic pain. A 9-year experience. J Neurosurg 70:519–524

26. Melzack R, Wall PD (1965) Pain mechanisms: a new theory. Science 150:1971–1979

27. Sciacca V, Mingoli A, di Marzo L, Fiume CMD, Cavallaro A (1989) Predictive value of transcutaneous oxygen tension measurement in the indication for spinal cord stimulation in patients with peripheral vascular disease: preliminary results. Vasc Surg 128–132

Authors' address:

Dr. med. L. Claeys
Academic Teaching Hospital Cologne-Porz
Dept. of General and Vascular Surgery
Urbacher Weg 19
D-51149 Cologne, FRG

Vascular disease and spinal cord stimulation

M. J. H. M. Jacobs

Vascular Surgeon, Department of Surgery, Academic Medical Center,
University of Amsterdam, The Netherlands

Vascular reconstructive surgery is the therapy of choice in patients with limb-threatening ischemia. Improved vascular techniques and an aggressive surgical approach have contributed to an increased foot salvage in patients with ischemic rest pain, non-healing ischemic ulcers, and gangrene. Nevertheless, patients remain in whom vascular surgery has no realistic chance of success despite technical progress, an aggressive surgical approach, and repeated reconstructions.

Alternative treatment modalities such as laser recanalization and percutaneous transluminal angioplasty have a limited role as sole treatment for patients with limb-threatening ischemia. Beneficial effects of lumbar sympathectomy have been reported especially in patients with a systolic ankle-to-brachial pressure index higher than 0.30. However, many patients with ischemic ulceration and rest pain have indices lower than 0.30, and it is inevitable that many of them finally face a major amputation.

Spinal cord stimulation is a medically accepted therapeutic modality for the control of chronic pain. Recently, spinal cord stimulation has also successfully been used for patients with ischemic rest pain. Strikingly, not only pain relief could be achieved but also healing of ischemic ulcers. This suggests that spinal cord stimulation improves the nutritional blood flow, a supposition that was confirmed in a recent study with the use of intravital video-microscopy.

The patients selected in the Academic Medical Center for spinal cord stimulation suffer from arteriosclerotic critical ischemia and are non-reconstructable, as demonstrated by selective digital subtraction angiography. Critical limb ischemia, as defined by the European consensus on critical ischemia, means that the patients have persistent ischemic pain at rest for at least 2 weeks requiring analgetics and a systolic ankle pressure <50 mmHg. Non-reconstructable means that there is no suitable artery available for reconstructive surgery, as demonstrated by selective angiography delineating the anatomy of the large vessels throughout the limb and the foot. Furthermore, if only ankle or foot arteries are available to bypass while an autogenous vein is absent, the case is regarded as non-reconstructable.

Implantation of the electrode and pulse generator is a minor surgical procedure, which is performed under local anesthesia. We usually give prophylactic antibiotic treatment for 24 h. Implantation of the electrode is done with the patient in an oblique position whereafter a small vertical incision is made parallel to the spinal column. Under biplanar fluoroscopic control, the electrode is introduced into the epidural space at the level of L3/L4 and is placed in the midline at about the level of T10. Subsequently, the electrode is connected to an external stimulator and causes paresthesia in the legs. The lead is then manipulated until the patient experiences pleasant paraesthesiae extending down into the painful foot. The lead is fixed to the thoracolumbar fascia to prevent migration. It is extremely important that the patient

"

experiences paresthesia in the ischemic foot and, if so, a pulse generator can be connected to the epidural electrode. The pulse generator is implanted in a subcostal subcutaneous pouch and connected to the electrode via the subcutaneous extension lead. Unipolar or bipolar stimulation can be performed with a changeable pulse width and frequency. The amplitude of the pulses can be adjusted depending on the patient's subjective feeling of comfortable paresthesia.

An alternative approach is external stimulation for several days as a screening period and, if clinically successful, connection and implantation of the pulse generator. In patients with rest pain and ulceration, the symptoms are caused by a threatened skin microcirculation and, hence, tissue damage. The problem in this end-stage ischemia is how to evaluate objectively the changes induced by the treatment. Systolic ankle pressure measurements at rest and after treadmill exercise are generally accepted as the best non-invasive method to document arterial obstruction of the lower extremities. More distally, flow and pressure information from the distal arterial system can be obtained by venous and photo-electric plethysmography. These macrocirculatory methods enable assessment of the global hemodynamics in a region.

Tissue oxygen pressure measurements, laser Doppler fluxmetry, and radio-isotope clearance techniques can be performed to study the cutaneous blood flow. In several studies, these techniques have been used to evaluate the effects of spinal cord stimulation on skin microcirculation. Patients with a subjective improvement showed a significantly enhanced skin microcirculatory perfusion. The evaluation of the treatment of ischemic rest pain and ulceration should ideally be done at the level from which the ischemic phenomena originates, i.e., the skin nutritional capillaries. Intravital capillary microscopy is a non-invasive method to study the morphological pattern of the microcirculation and it allows the measurement of the blood velocity in the skin capillaries, which specifically reflects the nutritional blood flow.

During recent years, we investigated the effects of spinal cord stimulation on the nutritive microcirculatory blood flow in 35 patients with ischemic rest pain and ulcers, who were submitted for amputation [1].

Capillary density and diameter and red blood cell velocity before and after arterial occlusion were assessed by capillary microscopy. After spinal cord stimulation, 28 patients claimed immediate relief of pain which could be confirmed by intravital capillary microscopy. Capillary density and the red cell velocity increased significantly. During the first year of follow-up, seven patients underwent amputation, Life-table analysis revealed a cumulative foot salvage of 80, 58, and 48 per cent after 1, 2, and 3 years respectively. In patients with continued pain relief and in whom ischemic ulcers healed, capillary microscopy showed maintenance of the microcirculatory blood flow. The microcirculatory parameters were significantly higher in responders than in non-responders.

In general, electrical stimulation of the afferent nervous system is a very effective way to treat pain. The mechanisms by which spinal cord stimulation exerts pain relief and improves the blood flow are still not clear. The observation that adequate pain relief correlates with improved capillary flow, suggests that pain inhibition releases the sympathetic reflex vasoconstriction, which is known to occur in response to pain. Linderoth [2] performed experimental studies and found results which favor the hypothesis that spinal cord stimulation produces a transitory suppression of sympathetically dependent vasoconstriction, resulting in an increased peripheral tissue perfusion and, secondarily, a relief of ischemic pain. However, there may exist several

154

components in the vasodilatory mechanism. At present, several studies indicate that spinal cord stimulation relieves rest pain and enhances the microcirculatory blood flow, thereby improving ulcer healing in patients with criticial limb ischemia. Several prospective randomized studies are in progress and will prove in the near future whether or not spinal cord stimulation is an acceptable modality in the treatment of critical limb ischemia.

References

1. Jacobs MJHM, Jörning PJG, Beckers RCY et al (1990) Foot salvage and improvement of microvascular blood flow as a result of epidural spinal cord electrical stimulation. J Vasc Surg 12:354–360
2. Linderoth B (1992) Dorsal column stimulation and pain: experimental studies of putative neurochemical and neurophysiological mechanisms. Thesis. Stockholm, Karolinska Institute

Author's address:

M.J.H.M. Jacobs, MD
Academic Medical Center
Vascular Department
G4–105
Meibergdreef 9
NL-1105 AZ Amsterdam
The Netherlands

Laser-Doppler fluxmetry (LDF) in patients treated by spinal cord stimulation (SCS)

V. Sciacca

Policlinico Umberto 1, Dept. of Surgery, University of Rome "La Sapienza", Rome, Italy

Today, spinal cord stimulation (SCS), introduced as a therapeutic modality for the control of chronic pain of different ethiologies [18, 29], is used as an alternative method of treating patients with cirtical limb ischemia (CLI) that is neither amenable to vascular reconstructions nor responsive to medical treatment [1, 3, 5, 6, 8, 9, 12, 14, 15, 21, 30].

The noninvasive techniques available for evaluating microvascular modifications caused by SCS are:

- dynamic capillary computerized microscopy (DCM),
- transcutaneous oxygen tension (TcPO$_2$), and
- laser-Doppler fluxmetry (LDF).

Recently, DCM has shown that, in patients with critical ischemia of the lower limbs, SCS recruits capillaries not perfused in the control situation and enhances skin blood flow (13).

TcPO$_2$, based on oxygen delivery measured by Clark's electrode, has been used for evaluating limb ischemia, providing an assessment of cutaneous perfusion [4] and vasomotor tone [24]. Moreover TcPO$_2$ has been applied with success to quantify the local metabolic conditions improved by SCS [25] and to predict the efficacy of SCS in patients with peripheral vascular disease [26].

Laser-Doppler fluxmetry (LDF)

The measurement principle is based on registration of refraction, reflection, and partial absorption of the emitted 2 mW He-Ne laser signal (wave length 780 nm – TSI Laserflo BPM, St. Paul, Minnesota, USA) in the tissue being examined. An output signal, in millivolts, is created which is proportional to the product of the number of moving cells and their mean velocity. The depth of penetration of the laser-Doppler signal is about 0.7 to 1 mm, such that a sample volume of one cubic mm can be examined. The output signal cannot be calibrated to absolute value of blood flow, but it is linear to the flux of blood cells (mostly erythrocytes) within the skin microcirculation. Consequently, LDF allows recording of relative changes of blood cell flux in a given volume of tissue that includes nutritional capillaries, microvascular arteriovenous anastomoses and subdermal plexuses.

The principles and the limits governing the measurements of skin blood flow by LDF have been described in detail elsewhere [2, 7, 16, 17, 19, 22, 23, 31, 32].

The purpose of this study was to evaluate by LDF the SCS microcirculatory modifications.

Patients and methods

LDF measurements were done in 30 patients (pts) submitted to SCS. The indication for SCS was CLI of the lower (13 pts: nine men, four women, mean age 73 years – Group A) and of the upper limbs (17 pts: 16 women, one man, mean age 47 years – Group B: 15 scleroderma with secondary Raynaud's, two with Raynaud's disease).

In Group A patients vascular reconstructive surgery or lumbar sympathectomy had been performed previously without satisfactory results and preoperative or intraoperative angiography showed arteries unsuitable for further reconstructive surgical attempts.Medical treatment was not effective and all patients had intolerable rest pain, four of them with non-healing ischemic ulcers (less than 3 sqcm in diameter). The first patient was treated 13 months previously and the last one 7 days previously (mean follow-up 8 months). Only monopolar SCS was used with the lead tip between D9 and D12 and its effectiveness was assured by paresthesias in the ischemic areas. Eleven patients has a 7 – 15 day testing period, while in two pts the complete system was inserted in one stage.

In Group B all patients had a 5-year or longer clinical history, were unresponsive to medical treatment, and presented Raynaud's phenomenon, pain associated with polyrathralgia, skin induration, edema of acral portions of the extremities, sclerodactyl, masklike face, esophageal dysfunction and lung fibrosis. Three patients had facial teleangectasia and in another three trophic ulcers were present. Increased pigmentation, vitiligo, and renal disease were seldom associated. The first patient had been treated with SCS 49 months before and the last one 15 days before (mean follow-up 30 months). Two patients had been previously (4 and 6 years respectively) submitted to cervical sympathectomy (one bilateral, one right). The final position of the lead tip was between C3 and C7: monopolar in 14 patients, bipolar in one patient, and tetrapolar in two patients. After a 7 – 15 day testing period the electrode was permanently implanted and connected to the subcutaneous multiprogrammable neurostimulator.

LDF measurements, in standard environmental conditions with the patient in supine position, were done on the dorsum of the foot in Group A patients and on the thenar or hypothenar eminence in Group B patients. LDF flux, velocity and volume were monitored with the probe heated at 42 °C and 45 °C during three 30-min consecutive phases: phase I pacemaker off for 12 h, phase II pacemaker on, phase III pacemaker off. All patients had simultaneous measurement of $TcPO_2$ vasodilation index ($TcPO_2$ 42 °C/$TcPO_2$ 45 °C) and in Group B at the end of phases I and II they performed the Valsalva maneuver to ascertain the sympathetic activity. Moreover, in Group B patients arterial and venous norepinephrine (NE) levels in picograms were measured by chromatography according to Goldstein (10) in phases I and II, sampling blood from the radial artery and from the brachial vein without tourniquet.

Student's paired *t*-test and chi square test were used for statistical analysis, considering the five LDF and $TcPO_2$ readings of the last 5 min in each phase at 42 ° and 45 °C.

Results

Group A

Clinical results were good in 11 patients, with immediate pain relief and healing or improving of ulcer in two patients. In two patients with ischemic lesions amputation was unavoidable during the follow-up.

In 11 responder patients LDF measurements demonstrated a statistically significant increase ($p < 0.005$) of flux and volume parameters in phases II and III, while velocity remained almost unchanged (Figs. 1, 2). The flux and volume increases were more evident at 42 °C because the microvascular tone at lower temperature was higher. The LDF flux difference between 42 ° and 45 °C were statistically significant only in phase I while in phases II and III the hyperthermic stimulus was unable to modify the flux.

TcPO$_2$ vasodilation index increased from 0.54 ± 0.14 in phase I to 0.73 ± 0.08 and 0.77 ± 0.09 respectively in phases II and III ($p < 0.005$).

A diabetic patient with unsatisfactory result presented an elevated TcPO$_2$ vasodilation index in phase I (0.65) that decreased to 0.62 in phases II and III.

Group B

In 14 patients (Br) SCS caused complete pain relief and the patients reported a warmer skin feeling, while three patients (Bnr) did not experience that and pain was

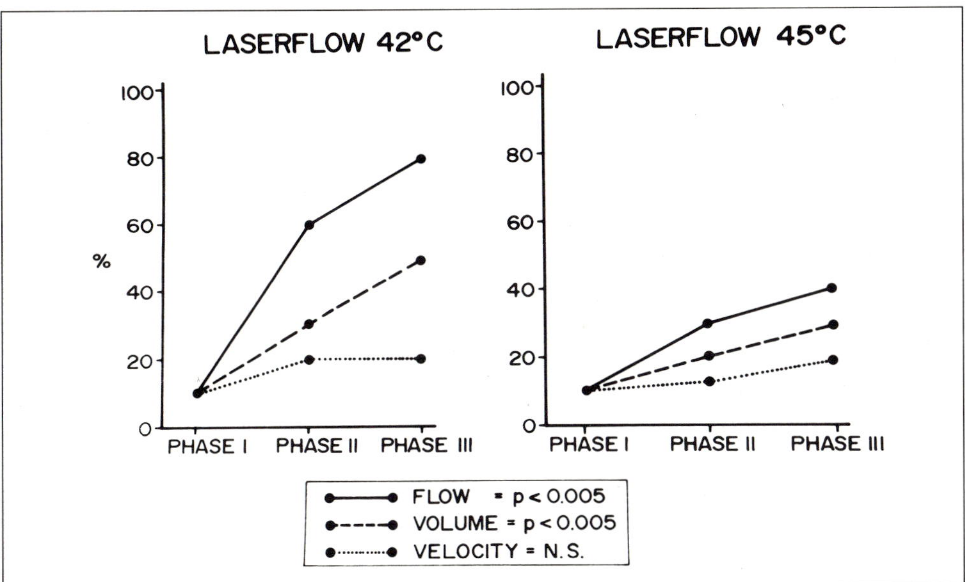

Fig. 1. Modifications of LDF parameters in phases I, II, and III. Notice that flux (= flow) and volume increase is more evident at 42 °C because the microvascular tone is higher

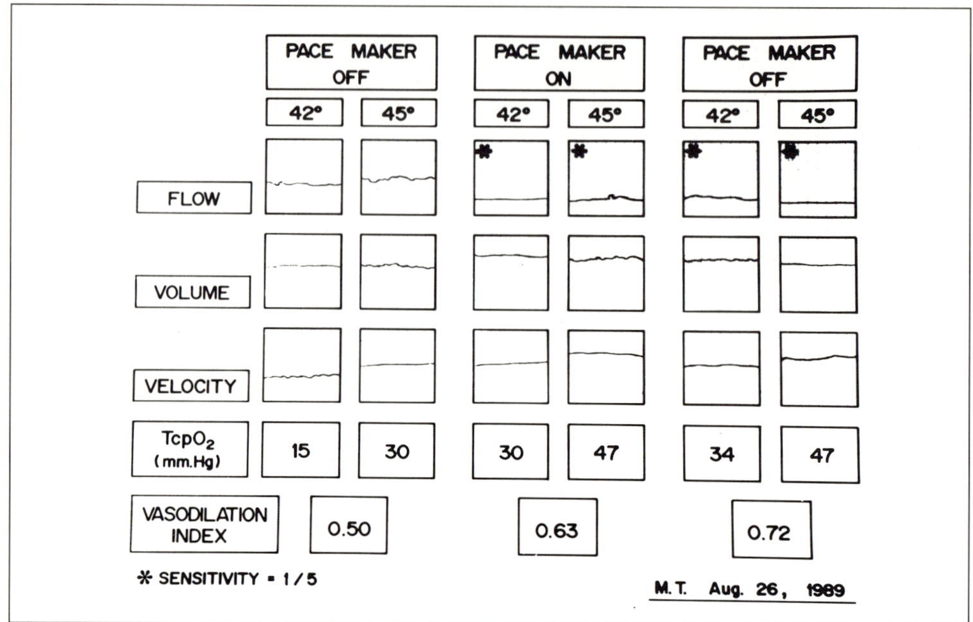

Fig. 2. LDF and TCPO$_2$ data in phases I, II, and III from a responder Group A patient. Notice that in phases II and III the scale sensitivity of flux (= flow) is 1/5 of the basal phase I tracing

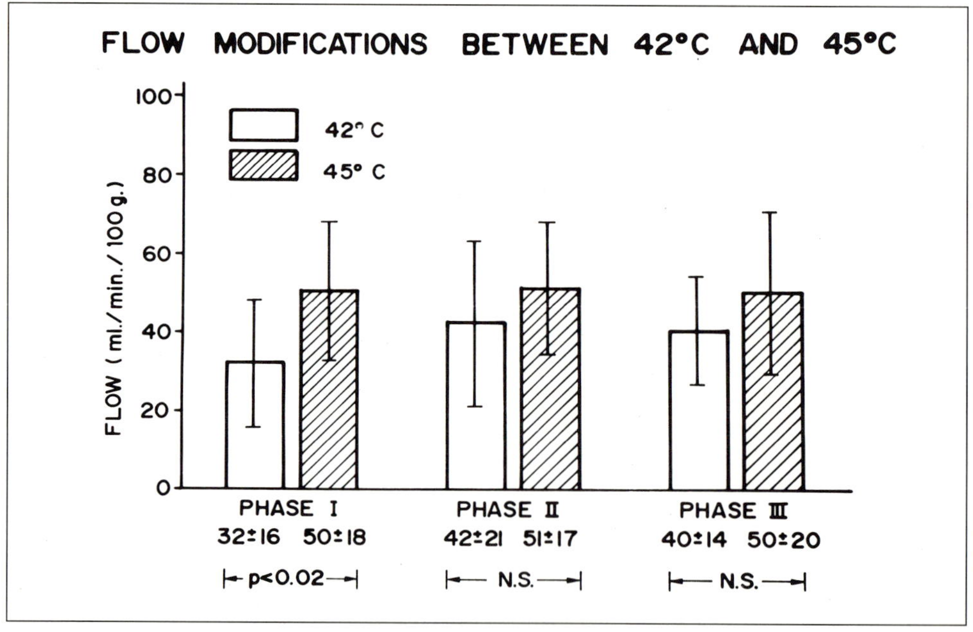

Fig. 3. Group B flux (= flow) modification between 42° and 45 °C significant only in phase I

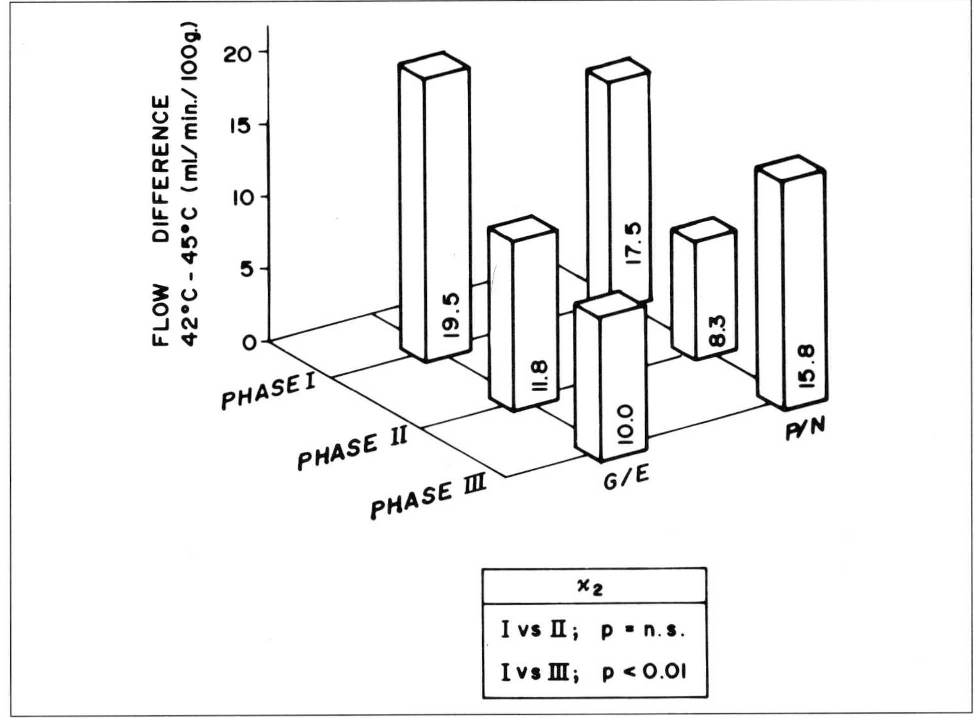

Fig. 4. Modifications of flux (= flow) difference in phases II and III. Notice the difference in phase III increases in nonresponder patients (G/E good/excellent results, P/N poor/null results)

relieved only partially. In the 14 responders there were decreases of edema, healing of the acral lesions and improvement of fingers' and lips' motility. LDF demonstrated a statistically significant flux increase between 42° and 45°C only in phase I ($p < 0.02$) while in phases II and III the hyperthermic stimulus did not modify the flux (Fig. 3). The flux differences between 42° and 45°C were statistically significant between the phases I and III only in the 14 responders (Br) (chi square: $p < 0.01$), (Fig. 4). LDF tracings during the Valslava maneuver whether the pacemaker was off or on showed normal decrease of flux in all patients excluding the two patients previously sympathectomized thus demonstrating a preserved sympathetic activity (Fig. 5). TcPO$_2$ vasodilation index increased from 0.39 ± 0.21 in phase I to 0.74 ± 0.15 and 0.73 ± 0.08 respectively in phases II and III ($p < 0.001$) in responder patients, testifying to a reduced vasomotor tone.

NE levels, available only in 12 patients for technical reasons, demonstrated an inversion of arteriovenous difference in seven of nine responders and in none of the nonresponders.

Discussion

From our experience LDF, coupled or not with TcPO$_2$, is an accurate non-invasive method of evaluating microcirculatory changes induced by SCS. LDF data from this

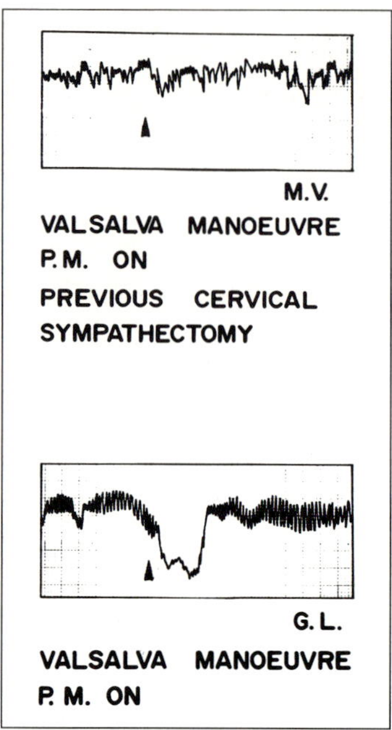

Fig. 5. LDF tracings during Valsalva maneuver. Notice the normal response in spite of the pacemaker's being on

study compare favorably with those reported by Jacobs et al. [13, 14] with DCM: they demonstrated an increase of capillary density, flow rate, and red blood cell velocity without significant capillary diameter modifications. The LDF volume increase, which influences LDF flux amelioration, represents the augmented back-scattered red blood cell signals and it matches well with the increased capillary density related to SCS reperfusion of inactive capillaries.

The increased $TcPO_2$ vasodilation index in phases II and III, coupled with the LDF modifications, testifies to a reduced vasomotor tone and supports the theory of decreased sympathetic activity caused by SCS [20, 27, 28], which lasted as well during the pacemaker switch off phase (III).

Moreover, the normal response to Valsalva maneuver demonstrates that the sympathetic fiber discharge is not completely abolished by SCS.

The presence of vasospastic microcirculatory disturbances, such as in primary or secondary Raynaud's phenomenon, with elevated vasomotor tone, represents the best indication to SCS when medical treatment is unsuccessful.

The NE level modification with arteriovenous ratio decrease, which usually occurs after surgical sympathectomy [11], has been observed in our SCS responders of Group B patients in whom LDF difference between 42° and 45 °C was significantly decreased and long lasting in phase III; this phenomenon suggests that SCS mechanism is a sort of neuromodulation with reversible functional electrical sympathicolysis [20]. The SCS effect in scleroderma patients seems to be mediated biochemically: the decreased NE release from sympathetic nerve endings ameliorates local microcirculatory (LDF) and, consequently, metabolic ($TcPO_2$) conditions.

The SCS efficacy in spite of a previous surgical sympathectomy suggests either an autonomic fiber regeneration or a different pathway of SCS stimuli.

162

Conclusions

We believe that LDF is an accurate, quick, and simple method of measuring microcirculatory modification in patients with SCS: it parallels the $TcPO_2$ and DCM modifications, but has the advantage of being less expensive and easier in comparison to the above-mentioned techniques.

References

1. Augustinsson, LE, Holm J, Carlsson CA et al (1985) Epidural electrical stimulation in severe limb ischemia. Evidence of pain relief, increased blood flow and a possible limb saving effect. Ann Surg 202:104−110
2. Braveman IM, Keh A, Goldminz D (1990) Correlations of laser Doppler wave patterns with underlying microvascular anatomy. J Invest Dermat 95:283−286
3. Broseta J, Barbara J, De Vera JA et al (1985) Spinal cord stimulation in peripheral arterial disease. J Neurosurg 64:71−80
4. Cina C, Katsamouris A, Megerman J et al (1984) Utility of transcutaneous oxygen tissue measurements in peripheral arterial occlusive disease. J Vasc Surg 1:362−371
5. Cook AW, Oygar A, Baggenstos O et al (1976) Vascular disease of the extremities. Electrical stimulation of spinal cord and posterior roots. NY State J Med 76:366−368
6. Dooley DM, Kasprak M (1976) Modification of blood flow to the extremities by electrical stimulation of the nervous system. South Med J 69:1309−1311
7. Fagrell B (1985) Dynamics of skin microcirculation in humans. J Cardiovasc Pharm 7 (Suppl 3):S53−S58
8. Fiume D, Palombi M, Sciacca V et al (1989) Spinal cord stimulation (SCS) in peripheral ischemic pain. Pace 12:698−704
9. Galley D, Elharrar C, Scheffer J et al (1989) Neurostimulation et pathologie vasculaire: interet therapeutique a propos de 49 patients. Coeur 20:35−44
10. Goldstein DS, Feuerstein GZ, Izzo JL et al (1981) Validity and reliability of liquid chromatography with electrochemical detection for measuring plasma levels or norepinephrine and epinephrine in man. Life Sci 28:467−475
11. Goldstein DS, Bonner RF, Zimlichman R (1986) Indices of sympathetic vascular innervation in sympathectomized patients. J Auton Nerv Syst 15:309−318
12. Graber NJ, Lifson A (1987) The use of spinal cord stimulation for severe limb threatening ischemia. A preliminary report. Ann Vasc Surg 1:345−349
13. Jacobs MJ, Jorning PJ, Joshi SR et al (1988) Epidural spinal cord electrical stimulation improves microvascular blood flow in severe limb ischemia. Ann Surg 207:179−183
14. Jacobs MJ, Jorning PJ, Beckers RC et al (1990) Foot salvage and improvement of microvascular blood flow as a result of epidural spinal and cord electrical stimulation. J Vasc Surg 12:354−360
15. Jivegard L, Augustinsson LE, Carlsson CA et al (1987) Long-term results by epidural spinal electrical stimulation (ESES) in patients with inoperable severe lower limb ischemia. Eur J Vasc Surg 1:345−349
16. Karanfillian R, Lynch TG, Lee BC et al (1984) The assessment of skin blood flow in peripheral vascular disease by laser-Doppler velocimetry. Amer Surg 50:641−648
17. Kvernebo K, Megerman J, Hamilton G et al (1989) Response of skin photoplethysmography, laser Doppler flowmetry and transcutaneous oxygen tensiometry to stenosis-induced reductions in limb blood flow. Eur J Vasc Surg 3:113−120
18. Long DH (1977) Electrical stimulation for control in pain. Arch Surg 112:884−888
19. Lukkari-Rautiarinen E, Lepantalo M, Pietila J (1989) Reproducibility of skin blood flow, perfusion pressure and oxygen tension measurements in advanced lower limb ischaemia. Eur J Vasc Surg 3:345−350
20. Meglio M, Cioni B, Dal Lago A et al (1981) Pain control and improvement of peripheral blood flow following epidural spinal cord stimulation. J Neurosurg 54:821−823

21. Mingoli A, Sciacca V, Tamorri M et al (1993) Clinical results of epidural spinal cord electrical stimulation in patients affected with limb-threatening chronic arterial obstructive disease. Angiology 44:21−25
22. Nilsson GE, Tenland T, Oberg PA (1980) A new instrument for continuous measurements of tissue blood flow by light beating spectroscopy. IEEE Trans Biomed Eng BME 27:12−19
23. Nilsson GE, Tenland T, Oberg PA (1980) Evaluation of a laser Doppler flowmeter for measurements of tissue blood flow. IEEE Trans Biomed Eng BME 27:597−604
24. Rooke TW, Hollier LH, Osmundson PJ (1987) The influence of sympathetic nerves on transcutaneous oxygen tension in normal and ischemic lower extremities. Angiology 38:400−410
25. Sciacca V, Tamorri M, Rocco M et al (1986) Modifications of transcutaneous oxygen tension in lower limb peripheral occlusive disease patients treated with spinal cord stimulation. It J Surg Sci 16:279−282
26. Sciacca V, Mingoli A, Di Marzo L et al (1989) Predictive value of transcutaneous oxygen tension measurement in the indication for spinal cord stimulation in patients with peripheral vascular disease: Preliminary results. Vasc Surg 23:128−132
27. Sciacca V, Mingoli A, Maggiore C et al (1991) Laser Doppler flowmetry and transcutaneous oxygen tension in patients with severe arterial insufficiency treated by epidural spinal cord electrical stimulation. Vasc Surg 25:165−170
28. Sciacca V, Vignotto F, Mingoli A et al (1992) Indices of sympathetic vascular innervation in scleroderma patients treated by epidural spinal cord electrical stimulation (ESES). Vasc Surg 26:457−463
29. Shealy CN, Mortimer JT, Reswick JB (1967) Electrical inhibition of pain by stimulation of the dorsal columns: Preliminary clinical report. Anest Analg (Cleve) 46:589−491
30. Tealdi DG, Signorelli M, DeNale A et al (1987) Epidural spinal electrical stimulation in the treatment of ischemic pain. Int Angiol 6:435−437
31. Winsor T, Haumschild DG, Winsor D et al (1987) Clinical application of laser Doppler flowmetry for measurement of cutaneous circulation in health and disease. Angiology 38:727−736
32. Winsor T, Haumschild DJ, Winsor D et al (1989) Influence of local and environmental temperatures on cutaneous circulation with the use of laser Doppler flowmetry. Angiology 40:421−428

Authors' address:

Prof. Dr. V. Sciacca
Associate Professor of Surgery
Policlinico Umberto I, Dept. of Surgery
University of Rome 'La Sapienza'
Via E. Duse 22
I-00197 Rome
Italy

Can spinal cord stimulation reduce the amputation rate in patients with critical limb ischemia?

P. Kasprzak, D. Raithel

Department of Vascular Surgery, Nuremberg Hospital, Nuremberg, FRG

Introduction

For patients with critical limb ischemia the best immediate results can be obtained by vascular reconstructions and direct revascularization of ischemic tissue. The results of direct revascularization below knee differ in the literature with a range between 25 to 80% of open bypasses or limb salvages after 5 years, depending on center, selection criteria, type of procedure as well as bypass material [3, 4, 6]. Generally, the more proximal reconstructions show better results versus the distal ones, as well as primary reconstructions versus secondary or autologous vein versus graft material.

In some patients with poor run-off, occluded below-knee reconstruction, missing autologous vein or who are in bad general condition an alternative method of treatment can be of special value.

If recompensation of the patient by the whole spectrum of conservative treatment shows no permanent effect, or especially in cases where ischemic pain cannot be successfully treated, an indication for implantation of a spinal cord stimulator (SCS) should be discussed.

The first epidural stimulation of the spinal cord was performed in 1967 by Schealy and Mortimer, and the effect of this on the improvement of peripheral perfusion was described in 1976 by Cook and Dooley [1, 2, 5].

Material and methods

Between 1988 and July 1993 we qualified 94 patients for implantation of the SCS-device in the Department of Vascular Surgery in Nuremberg. There were 56 men and 38 women with a mean age of 68.9 years (27 – 87). The etiology of the distal occlusive disease was arteriosclerosis in 92 patients and thrombangitis in the two youngest. Out of 92 arteriosclerotic lesions the indication for neurostimulation was in 42 due to critical limb ischemia primarily, this means without a prior attempt of direct revascularization of distal arteries (27 in stage III, and 15 in stage IV after Fontaine). In 50 patients, a vascular reconstruction distal to the inguinal ligament, usually with a late bypass occlusion, had been carried out prior to the implantation of SCS. In this last group, the indication was an extreme short walking distance of serveral meters despite failing rest pain in 4, stage III in 28, and state IV in 18 patients. In 46 patients (48.9%) pathologic glucose levels were found. Eight of these patients (8.5%) were without treatment, 24 (25.5%) received oral medication, and 14 (14.9%) were on insulin. The implantation of SCS device (Itrel Metronic) was carried out under local anesthesia, and an epidural electrode was placed at the level of Th 11 −Th 12 under x-ray monitoring, usually in a midline position. The intraoperative test stimulation was decisive for the level of electrode placement.

The electrode and pulse generator can be implanted either simultaneously or in stage procedure. In a stage procedure an implantation of an electrode is followed by a 5 − 7-day period of test stimulation with a final implantation of the pulse generator only in responding patients. This kind of procedure was carried out in six patients. Only in one of these patients no effect was observed during the 1-week test phase. In the same patient no intraoperative effect of stimulation has been seen either. In another six patients, a trial of electrode implantation alone was carried out. In two of these patients the electrode could not be inserted epidurally due to technical problems (in patients who had undergone prior spinal cord surgery). Two patients reported severe back pain during intraoperative stimulation, so that the electrode could not be placed. In two patients no proper response was possible due to cerebral sclerosis (no compliance). Simultaneous procedures were carried out in 82 patients (87.2%) with an implantation of the electrode and the pulse generator at the same time. The precondition for a one-stage implantation is the positive intraoperative test stimulation with setting off the stimuli in the area of the relevant extremity and on the level of the usual pain, respectively in the area of ulcerations and necroses. The advantages of simultaneous stimulation are a shorter hospital stay as well a lower likeliness of infection, especially in patients with stage IV. On the other hand, the stage procedure was of special value at the beginning of the implantation as well as considering the high cost of the implanted devices.

Early results

The perioperative early results refer to a 30-day complication and mortality rate, although the majority of the patients could be dismissed after a 1- to 2-week stay. The perioperative mortality rate was 2.1%. One patient died due to specific complications of implantation (meningitis), another patient died due to myocardial infarction 2 weeks post implantation and after discharge from the clinic. The complication rate was 9.6% (nine patients). In one patient a meningitis was observed, which led to the death of the patient despite electrode explanation and treatment. In another five patients an SCS explantation or correction was necessary during the first 30 days. The amputation rate during the first 30 days was 4.3% (in four patients a major amputation such as forefoot, lower limb or upper limb had to be carried out). Toe amputations had to be regarded as part of the therapy − in our opinion, and they were not included in the amputation rates.

Late results

During the follow-up of a minimum of 3 months up to 5 years, the course of all patients could be followed referring to clinical results, possible vascular reconstructions, amputation frequency and morbidity. The average follow-up totalled 24 months. The number of patients who were followed for a minimum of 20 months amounted to 36, and a life-table analysis was possible only for 2 years postoperatively due to an insufficient number of patients at risk after 3 years. Surgical correction

166

of SCS was necessary in 13 patients (13.8%), including electrode corrections in displaced electrodes, electrode or extension cord fractions, and generator exchange. In four patients an SCS explantation was carried out due to infections; in one other patient the pulse generator had perforated through the skin with subsequent infection, but the device could be saved by implantation on the contralateral side while maintaing SCS function. In summary, septic complications were observed in five patients (5.3%). A non-working device was explanted in four other patients (4.3%). All in all, 14 patients did not show any SCS function (six implantation trials, four explantations due to infections and four explantations due to failing function). A success of the operation, meaning a healing of stage IV including successful toe amputations and improvement of the patient from stage III to stage II, was observed in 61 patients (64.9%). This number includes the four patients with bypass occlusion and extremely short walking distance. In all of them a prolonging of the walking distance up to several hundred meters was reached. No benefit of SCS stimulation was found in 12 patients (12.8%). Twenty-one patients had to undergo major amputation (forefoot, lower limb or upper limb), equivalent to a frequency of 22.3%. During follow-up 20 patients died (21.3%). The time of amputation as well as the mortality rate of patients can be drawn from Figure 1 (one patient who died 4 years after implantation is not included in the table).

During follow-up five of the 21 amputated patients died (23.8%), as did 15 of the 73 who had not undergone any amputation (20.5%), so that no significant difference could be found in the mortality rate with or without amputation. Postoperatively a total of 10 patients had to undergo a distal vascular reconstruction due to a persistent critical limb ischemia. Six of them had a working SCS, and four had a non-implanted or explanted SCS. The numbers of the patients as well as the amputation rate can be drawn from Tables 1 and 2.

The interpretation of these data is difficult due to the fact that the number of patients in three of the four groups is small. However, there is a clear impression of a non-varying amputation rate in the groups with functioning SCS (n = 74 and n = 6), as well as in groups without SCS (n = 10 and n = 14) independent of a further bypass operation.

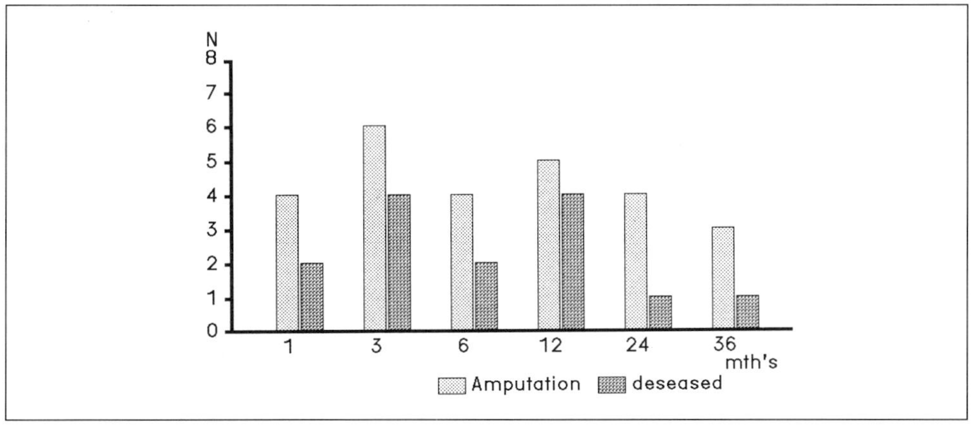

Fig. 1. Amputations/mortality in months after SCS implantation

Table 1. Additional distal vascular reconstruction for SCS in function (+) and SCS not implanted or explanted (−)

	No additional reconstruction	Additional reconstruction
SCS +	74	6
SCS −	10	4

Table 2. Major amputations for SCS (+) and SCS (−) and additional vascular reconstructions

	No additional reconstruction	Additional reconstruction
SCS +	14 (18.9%)	1 (16.7%)
SCS −	4 (40%)	2 (50%)

This impression is backed by judgment of SCS implantations after an average of 20 months and excluding the 10 patients who had received a bypass. In the remaining 84 patients successful regrading of patients back to stage II was possible in 55 patients (65.5%), no benefit was seen in 11 patients (13.1%), and amputation was necessary in 18 (21.4%). Judging the patients depending on primary SCS implantation compared to implantation of an SCS after occlusion of a vascular reconstruction, patients with primary SCS implantation showed a lower amputation rate than patients with SCS implantation after bypass occlusion. The highest amputation rate was observed in patients with an advanced state IV (Table 3).

The question of indication for SCS implantation in patients with diabetes mellitus cannot be clearly answered due to our patient population. We could only observe a trend that good results could be seen in patients with no diabetes (71%) compared to 62% in orally treated patients, 57% in insulin patients, and 50% in pathologic glucose test without treatment. As far as the amputation rate is concerned, we found a higher rate of 38% or 36% in the group of non-treated and insulin patients compared to the group of non-diabetics and orally treated patients with 17 or 21%, respectively.

The main question about a possible reduction of the amputation rate with the help of SCS implantation can be answered only by comparing the 80 implanted and working SCS devices with the 14 patients with a attempt of implantation or explanted SCS. Comparing these two groups, we found that in the group with working SCS

Table 3. Amputations (% of patients at risk) in groups (indication/year)

Year (n)	88 (1)	90 (7)	91 (32)	92 (34)	93 (20)
III				1 (10%)	1 (11%)
IV			2 (50%)	2 (25%)	
II (BP occl.)					
III (BP occl.)			3 (30%)	2 (25%)	
IV (BP oocl.)		2 (67%)	6 (60%)	1 (33%)	

a major amputation had to be carried out in 15 patients, that being equivalent to an amputation rate of 18.8%. In the patients with non-implanted or explanted SCS the amputation rate was significantly higher, namely, 42.9% (6 out of 14). Unfortunately, despite that the indication was similar in both groups, the follow-up is different with 441 vs. 661 days, so that another comparison has to be carried out.

Up through December 31, 1991, 40 SCS were implanted, which is equivalent to 43% of all patients. Out of these 40 SCS, 29 were functioning and 11 had to be given up or had to be explanted early. The indication for implantation was similar in both groups. Out of this patient group 13 had to undergo amputation during follow-up, which is equivalent to about 62% of all amputations. The follow-up for both patient groups is comparable to 712 days of working SCS devices and 739 days for patients without SCS. Major amputations were necessary in eight of the 29 patients with working SCS, that being equivalent to an amputation rate of 27.6% after 2 years compared to five out of 11 patients without SCS, which is equivalent to an amputation rate of 45.5% after two years, too. Finally, the question whether the amputation rate (major amputations) in patients with critical limb ischemia could be reduced by implantation of an SCS device can be answered with "yes". However, there are limits for these findings. First, there are the questions of indication and the timing of the operation which have to be considered. The results of SCS in instable lesions, early occlusions of bypasses as well as in large necroses are significantly worse than in patients who undergo operation because of stable and distal lesions or rest pain in an elective stage. There is still a need for further research considering the influence of polyneuropathy referring to diabetes mellitus, in order to be able to correctly judge the results of this therapy. The missing compliance, for example in cerebral scleroris, is another reason for the limits of a successful treatment of patients with critical limb ischemia by implantation of an SCS. The positive impressions gained after implantation of an SCS device outweigh the disadvantages, although many questions cannot be answered before an exact evaluation of the microcirculation in comparison to clinical data will be carried out in a prospective randomized study.

References

1. Cook AW, Oygar A, Baggenstos P et al. (1976) Vascular disease of the extremities: electrical stimulation of the spinal cord and the posterior roots. NY State J Med 76:366−368
2. Dooley D, Kasprak M (1976) Modifications of blood flow to the extremities by electrical stimulation of the nervous system. South Med J 69:1309−1311
3. Feinberg RL, Winter RP, Wheeler JR et al. (1990) The use of composite grafts in femorocrural bypasses performed for limb salvage: A review of 108 consecutive cases and comparison with 57 in situ saphenous vein bypasses. J Vasc Surg 12:257−263
4. Kikta MJ, Preston Flanigan D, Bishara RA et al. (1987) Long-term follow-up of patients having infrainguinal bypass performed below stenotic but hemodynamically normal aortoiliac vessels. J Vasc Surg 5:319−328
5. Shealy CN, Mortimer JT, Reswick JB (1978) Electrical inhibition of pain by stimulation of the dorsal columns: Preliminary clinical report. Anest Analg 46:489−491
6. Wengerter KR, Veith FJ, Gupta SK et al. (1990) Influence of vein size (diameter) on infrapopliteal reversed vein graft patency. J Vasc Surg 11:525−531

Authors' address:

Dr. med. P. Kasprzak, Abt. für Gefäßchirurgie, Klinikum Nürnberg, Zentrum für Chirurgie Flurstr. 17, D-90419 Nürnberg, FRG

Clinical studies

ESES-trial: Evaluation of epidural spinal cord electrical stimulation (ESES) in critical limb ischemia — a randomized controlled clinical trial

H. M. Klomp[1], G. H. J. J. Spincemaille[2], E. W. Steyerberg[3], M. Y. Berger[3], J. D. F. Habbema[3], H. van Urk[1] for the ESES study group

[1]University Hospital Rotterdam-Dijkzigt, Department of General Surgery, Vascular Unit, Rotterdam, The Netherlands,
[2]De Wever Hospital, Department of Neurosurgery, Heerlen, The Netherlands,
[3]Erasmus University Rotterdam, Center for Clinical Decision Sciences, Rotterdam, The Netherlands

Introduction

Peripheral arterial disease due to atherosclerosis is a common disease, particularly among the elderly. The prevalence of symptoms of intermittent claudication was reported to be 0.2–1.9% for men below 50 years old, rapidly rising with age to as high as 10.4% in age groups 60–90 [6]. Clinical progress to more severe degrees of ischemia will occur in about a quarter of these patients and in about 10% to limb-threatening ischemia [9]. In population-based studies the incidence of amputation in patients who had developed claudication was reported to be 1.6–1.8% [7]. Adverse prognostic factors for limb survival include advanced age, distal vessel disease, rest pain, continuing smoking, and diabetes. In the literature on the natural history of critical ischemia, this condition is considered to have a poor prognosis leading to amputation of the limb in 60–80% of patients within a year. Despite major advances in limb salvage by vascular repair, there remain limbs for which a revascularization (re)intervention is not appropriate. Until recently, the treatment of patients with critical ischemia of the lower extremities, in whom vascular reconstructive procedures are impossible or deemed unsuccessful, was restricted to conservative treatment. Ischemic pain is treated with analgesics, vasoactive medication may lead to some improvement of (micro)circulation, and ischemic skin lesions require local wound care. Ultimately, however, these patients face a major amputation.

A number of studies has been carried out to evaluate the use of Epidural Spinal cord Electrical Stimulation (ESES) for ischemia of the leg, leading to enthusiastic recommendation of this treatment [1–5, 8, 10, 11, 13, 16]. One-year limb survival was reported to be about 80%, 2-year survival about 50%. However, most studies were uncontrolled or made historical comparisons. The best information on whether

The ESES study group:
H. A. van Dijk, P. J. Theuvenet, R. J. van Det, P. de Smit, H. E. van de Aa, J. J. A. M. van den Dungen, M. J. Staal, N. A. J. J. du Bois, A. I. Veeger, T. I. Yo, G. Kazemier, C. H. A. Wittens, J. Lens, A. G. M. Hoofwijk, J. C. Sier, N. Lambooy, A. C. van der Ham, M. A. Wicks, E. A. Kole, F. J. N. A. Simons, J. Buth, H. P. J. K. M. van Houtte, A. J. Mulder, F. Bal, F. L. Moll, E. Scholten, A. L. Liem, J. H. M. Tordoir, M. van Kleef, T. H. A. Bikkers, M. J. H. M. Jacobs, D. Ubbink, D. van Lent, P. J. van Elk, A. H. Wigboldus
Grant: Sickness Funds Council (Health Insurance Board). The Netherlands

ESES reduces the incidence of amputation and does more good than harm to patients with severe ischemia of the lower extremity is generated by a randomized controlled clinical trial (RCCT). In this paper, we describe the design and progress of the ESES-trial in the Netherlands.

Designs issues

Trial design: The study is set up as a randomized controlled clinical trial. The treatment strategies: ESES, if necessary supplement by conservative treatment, and optimal conservative treatment are allocated at random to patients that meet the inclusion criteria. Eighteen centers collaborate in the study. All patient data are collected on highly standardized patient-record-forms in the form of a booklet.

Objectives: The aim of the trial is to compare "ESES-treatment" with conservative treatment, referred to as "standard treatment", in patients with non-reconstructible critical ischemia of a leg. Both treatments will be analyzed with regard to patient survival, limb survival and health state, in relation to the involved cost over a time-period of at least 18 months.

Pragmatic set up: We decided that the primary question that needs to be answered is whether the decision to give ESES-treatment would improve the subsequent health of a patient more than the decision to give standard treatment. In this study a comparison is made of the two treatments under the conditions in which they would be applied in clinical practice. The approach is thus pragmatic and aims at answering the question, which mode of therapy works best rather than how it works [15].

Outcomes: In the condition of non-reconstructible critical ischemia effectiveness of treatment cannot be expressed in so-called "hard" endpoints only. Research reports in vascular surgery generally focus on mortality, limb survival, and complications, whereas the patients' subjective feelings and quality of life are very important aspects of the patients' clinical condition, affecting the decision whether or not to perform a therapeutical procedure [17]. The ideal outcome would be the patients' health for his remaining life. In critical ischemia salvation of the limb is an important endpoint, but only in combination with an acceptable level of pain and discomfort.

We should also realize that, in addition to the "true effects" of the treatments studied, there will be psychosomatic effects, analogous to placebo effects. Whereas in this study the psychosomatic effects cannot be equalized between the two groups of patients (a nonfunctional device should be implanted in patients with standard treatment, which is ethically unacceptable), we include these within the "true effects" and assess psychosocial effects as results as well [15, 17]. Deferral of amputation can be considered a positive result, if based on an improved condition of the extremity and on an improved health state, additionally taking into account the short life expectancy of the group of patients studied.

If the condition of the limb becomes progressively worse, the vascular surgeon has to decide whether to amputate. The decision to amputate is taken on the following grounds:

- progressive tissue loss;
- intractable infection of ulceration or gangrene;
- explicit wish of the patient because of unbearable pain.

174

Primary outcome measures:
1) Health state
   a) patient survival
   b) limb survival
   c) quality of life (Nottingham Health Profile)
   d) pain (McGill Pain Questionnaire, visual analogue scales).
2) Cost effectiveness.

Secondary outcome measures:
1) Use of analgesics
2) Healing of ischemic skin lesions
3) Amputation level
4) Mobility (sub-module of the Sickness Impact Profile)
5) Complications
6) Macro- and microcirculatory measurements (Doppler ankle pressure, transcutaneous oximetry, diode laser Doppler fluxmetry, capillary microscopy)
7) Prognostic factors.

Pilot study: During 1989, in a pilot study in seven hospitals in the Netherlands 37 patients with critical ischemia were randomized, 18 to conservative treatment, 19 to spinal cord stimulation. Three patients died, the limb survival at one year in the conservative treatment group was 31%, and 65% in the ESES treatment group (with a mean follow-up of about 9 months). Trial schedules, data handling, registration forms, and health and pain questionnaires were tested.

Size of the trial: The sample size of the trial was assessed according to the estimated difference in limb survival between the ESES and standard treatment group. Median control survival was estimated at 6 months and median treated survival at 12 months, corresponding with a hazard ratio of 2. Assuming a total proportion of endpoints of 60%, a two-sided confidence level $(1-\alpha)$ of 95% and power (β) of 80%, about 120 patients are required in the trial (at least 56 patients per treatment arm).

Methods

Recruitment into the ESES-trial: From November 1991, all patients with critical limb ischemia seen by vascular surgeons in 18 participating hospitals in the Netherlands, in whom no meaningful vascular reconstructive procedure was possible, have been screened for eligibility for the ESES-trial. The surgeon explains the aims and procedures of the study. In addition, the patient receives written information. If the patient gives provisional consent, the baseline assessment is started and inclusion and exclusion criteria are checked. Those not excluded are given the opportunity to ask questions about the study and their written consent is then sought. The planned progress through the study is outlined in Fig. 1.

Eligibility: In order to accurately define the study group, a number of criteria were formulated, which inoperable patients with chronic, obliterating vascular disease must satisfy for participation in the study. These criteria were designed according to the "European Consensus Document on Critical Limb Ischemia" (March 1989). Specific inclusion criteria and exclusion criteria are listed in Table 1. If all in-

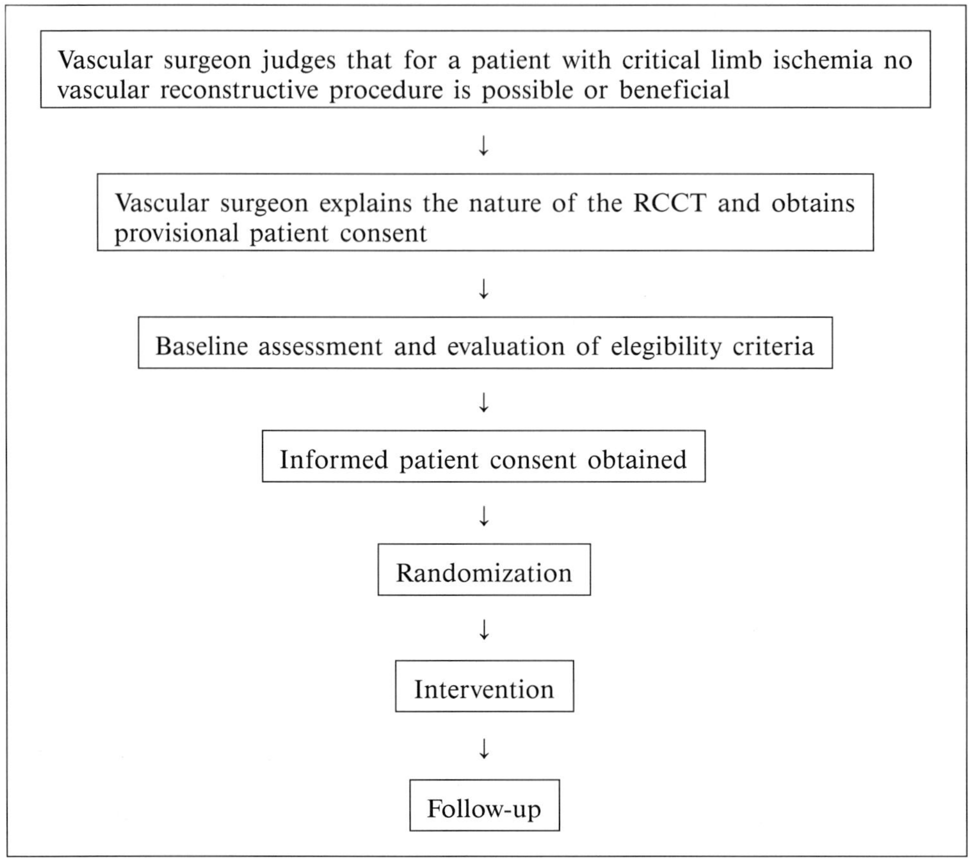

Fig. 1. Flow chart of patient progress through the ESES-trial

clusion criteria are met and none of the exclusion criteria, the patient is eligible to enter the trial.

There has always been a lot of discussion about the definition of critical limb ischemia, but this issue has become very prominent since Tompson et al. [14] presented data on 148 severely ischemic limbs of non-diabetic patients, presenting with rest pain, tissue necrosis or a combination of these. Fifty-one percent of these limbs had an ankle pressure > 50 mmHg. Furthermore, the results showed that a higher ankle pressure did not correspond with a better prognosis. Therefore, from March 1993 on we also included patients with ankle pressures 50 – 70 mmHg as a separate stratum in treatment allocation.

Treatment allocation: In this multi-center trial, treatment allocation is centralized in an independent research assistance institute. The clinician phones the randomization center, which step-by-step checks eligibility, registers the patient and gives the treatment assignment right away, using a computer program. The randomization method is stratified randomization as described by Zelen [18]. Strata are formed by presence or absence of diabetes, institution, and inclusion by the original or expanded criteria.

176

Table 1. ESES-trial inclusion and exclusion criteria

Inclusion Criteria:
  Critical ischemia of one of the lower limbs in patients, for whom a meaningful vascular reconstructive procedure is considered not to be possible:
  1 a. Persistent rest pain for at least 2 weeks, being treated with analgesics,
    b. and/or ulceration or gangrene of foot or toes.
  2 a. Systolic ankle pressure using Doppler ultrasound less than 50 mmHg or ankle-brachial-index (ABI) less than 35%.
    b. For patients with diabetes and incompressible vessels, as a result of which ankle pressure cannot be reliably measured: absence of arterial ankle pulsations.
  3. Patient informed consent.

Exclusion Criteria:
  1. Vascular disorders other than atherosclerotic disease.
  2. No rest pain (e.g., only intermittent claudication) and no ulceration or gangrene.
  3. Ankle pressure >50 mmHg or ABI >35%, when these pressures can be reliably measured.
  4. Palpable ankle pulsations in patients with diabetes and incompressible vessels.
  5. Ulceration deeper than the fascia or with largest diameter >3 cm.
  6. Infected, suppurating gangrene or gangrene with largest diameter >3 cm.
  7. Intractable infection of ulceration or gangrene.
  8. Critical ischemia of both legs.
  9. Possibility of a meaningful vascular reconstruction.
  10. Neoplastic or other disease with a life expectancy <1 year.
  11. Presence of a cardiac pacemaker.
  12. Impossibility to implant an epidural electrode and stimulator.
  13. Previous participation in an ESES-trial or pilot study.
  14. Psychosocial incompetence of the patient to satisfy the follow-up schedule.

Treatment regimes: Those patients who are allocated to standard treatment receive analgesics, peripheral vasoactive drugs, local wound treatment and antibiotics, if necessary. There is a list of recommended medication, but there is no fixed treatment regimen. The clinician should, in particular, aim at adequate pain suppression. As in chronic pain, continuous pain suppression is advised, so that analgesics will have to be given several times a day. If necessary, narcotic analgesics will be used.

Those allocated to ESES treatment will additionally receive an implantable spinal cord stimulation system (Itrell II IPG and Quad lead). In all participating centers a neurosurgeon or anesthesiologist is acquainted with the implantation technique. The lead is placed in the epidural space and manipulated until the patient experiences pleasant paresthesia extending down into the painful area. The lead and pulse generator are implanted during the same session. The settings of the system can be adjusted in the outpatient clinic. Again, one should aim at adequate pain suppression.

If pain suppression is inadequate, the effect should be optimized by altering the stimulation setting. Pain medication should be supplemented. Insufficient effect of ESES on the pain is to be expected in about 15% of the patients treated. In case of technical problems, electrode migration or infection, attempts should be made to resolve the difficulties (by replacing or repositioning electrode or stimulator or treating with antibiotics). Clinical treatment may be necessary. When all moves to correct such problems fail, the system will be explanted. The patient is analyzed in the original group, but receives standard treatment.

	Vascular surgeon (standard and ESES)				Neurosurg. (ESES)	Coord. center
	Exam	Qu	Dop	μc	Stim	Qu
Intake	±	±	±	±	+	
t = 0 randomization						
1 month	±		±	±	+	±
3 months	±		±	±	+	±
6 months	±		±	±	+	±
12 months	±		±	±	+	±
18 months	±		±	±	+	±
end of study	±				+	

Abbreviations used: ± = ESES treatment and standard treatment groups; + = applies only to ESES treatment group; Exam = clinical examination; Qu = questionaire: pain score, Nottingham Health Profile; Dop = Doppler ankle pressure measurement; μc = microcirculatory measurements; stim = follow-up stimulation settings by neurosurgeon or anesthesiologist

Fig. 2. Flow chart of follow-up

In case of unbearable pain in which the patient requests amputation, the clinician checks whether treatment has been maximized. If a patient refuses to continue with the allocated treatment, then in case of ESES treatment the stimulator must be explanted. The patient will be followed up, receiving standard treatment. When it concerns a patient allocated to standard treatment, follow-up will also be continued, irrespective of the policy to be pursued.

Follow up: To evaluate the clinical course, the patients are followed up for at least 18 months by the vascular surgeons who entered them in the trial. The follow-up flow chart is drawn in Fig. 2. The check-ups at the neurosurgeon or anesthesiologist, which are only relevant to patients who received ESES-treatment, include the effect of stimulation, registration of the setting, and possible technical or clinical complications.

The intake questionnaire about quality-of-life and pain has to be completed by the patient before randomization. The coordination center mails the follow-up questionnaires to the patient's home 2–4 weeks after each follow-up visit; a stamped reply envelope is provided. The measurement of general well-being and pain takes place between two follow-up visits to minimize the effect of follow-up visits and differences in data collection between ESES and standard treatment. The quality-of-life instrument is the Dutch translation of the Nottingham Health Profile (NHP). The NHP is aimed at measuring changes in behavior and activities that the patient relates to his state of health. Pain is quantified using visual analogue scales and the McGill pain questionnaire.

Organization: The study is set up as a multi-center trial with local responsibility. In the coordination center in the University Hospital Rotterdam-Dijkzigt, the trial-coordinator and the administrative assistent receive the original case-record-forms and patient questionnaires, check and process all data, maintain a concurrent database, monitor the progress and quality of the trial, and give information to participants. Within each clinic a center-coordinator is responsible for the care of trial-patients. Further involved in the organization of the trial are a project-manager, a data-manager, a statistician, and an epidemiologist. An independent research assistance institute in Amsterdam performs the randomization procedure. The ethical committee and the steering committee supervise trial conduct and progress.

Analysis: Efficacy and safety as regards clinical events will be analyzed according to the intention-to-treat principle, i. e. incorporating all randomized patients who fulfilled the inclusion criteria. There will be no interim-analysis.

Economic evaluation: The alternative treatments are being compared in terms of opportunity costs per patient. The costs can be classified into direct medical costs (inside and outside the hospital), direct not-medical costs (patient costs), and indirect costs. The volume of procedures will be determined for all patients, while the cost per procedure will be estimated in a sample. Important determinants will be in-hospital stay, operative procedures, and rehabilitation.

Results

Accrual rate: The estimated accrual rate turned out to be lower than expected, even though we estimated very cautiously. Randomization started in November 1991, and until July 1993, 90 patients were enrolled in the trial. There has been quite some variation as regards the number of recruited patients among the clinics, two hospitals providing over 30% of all patients. The intake rate is summarized in Fig. 3.

Baseline characteristics: A number of intake data on 88 patients is listed in Table 2. Calculating the total number of previous intervention procedures for the critically ischemic limb studied, a mean of 2.3 interventions was performed: 14 limbs no intervention (16%), 24 limbs one intervention (27%), 18 limbs two interventions (20%), 13 limbs three interventions (15%) and 19 limbs four or more interventions (22%).

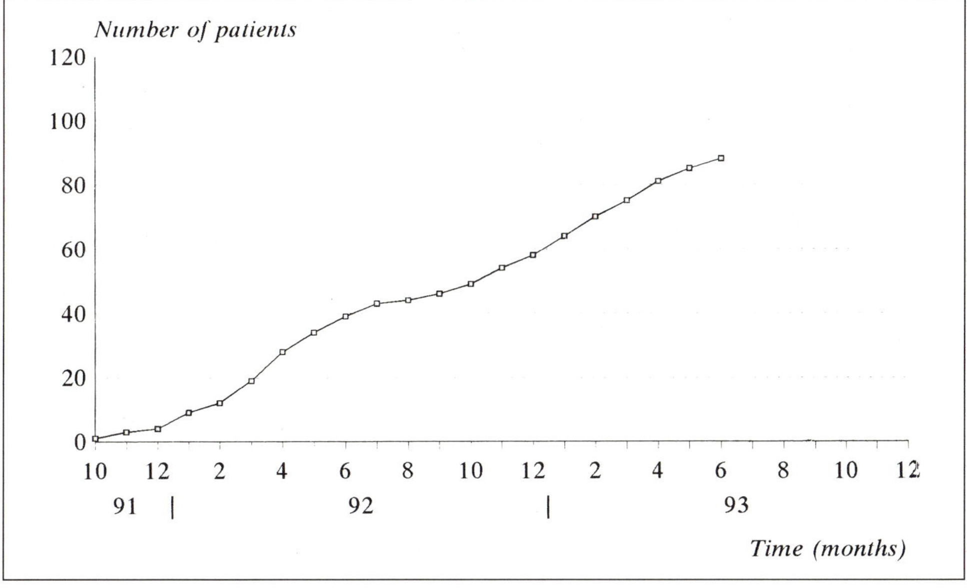

Fig. 3. Intake ESES-trial

Table 2. Baseline characteristics on 88 patients enrolled in the ESES-trial

	frequency	%	
Male (mean age)	58	66	(70 yr)
Female (mean age)	30	34	(76 yr)
Diabetes	37	42	
insulin dependent	17	19	
Rest pain	87	99	
Ischemic skin lesions	56	64	
Contralateral limb:			
asymptomatic	40	45	
symptomatic	36	41	
amputated	12	14	
Smoking:			
never	25	28	
stopped >1 yr	25	28	
smoking	38	43	
Myocardial infarction in history	30	34	
Angina pectoris	16	18	
CVA	10	11	
TIA	10	11	

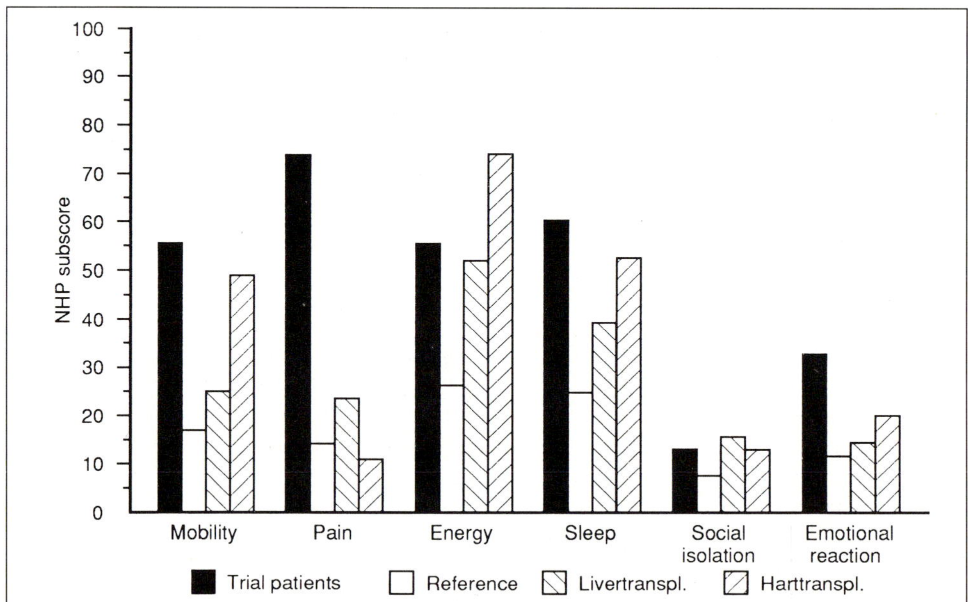

Fig. 4. Baseline quality-of-life score of trial-patients as compared to reference values and scores of patients on waiting list for liver transplantation resp. heart transplantation

The mean ankle pressure in non-diabetic patients was 42 mmHg, the mean ankle-brachial pressure index was 25%.

Quality of life: We compared the baseline quality-of-life score of the trial patients with reference values matched on age and sex, taken from a random sample of 2173

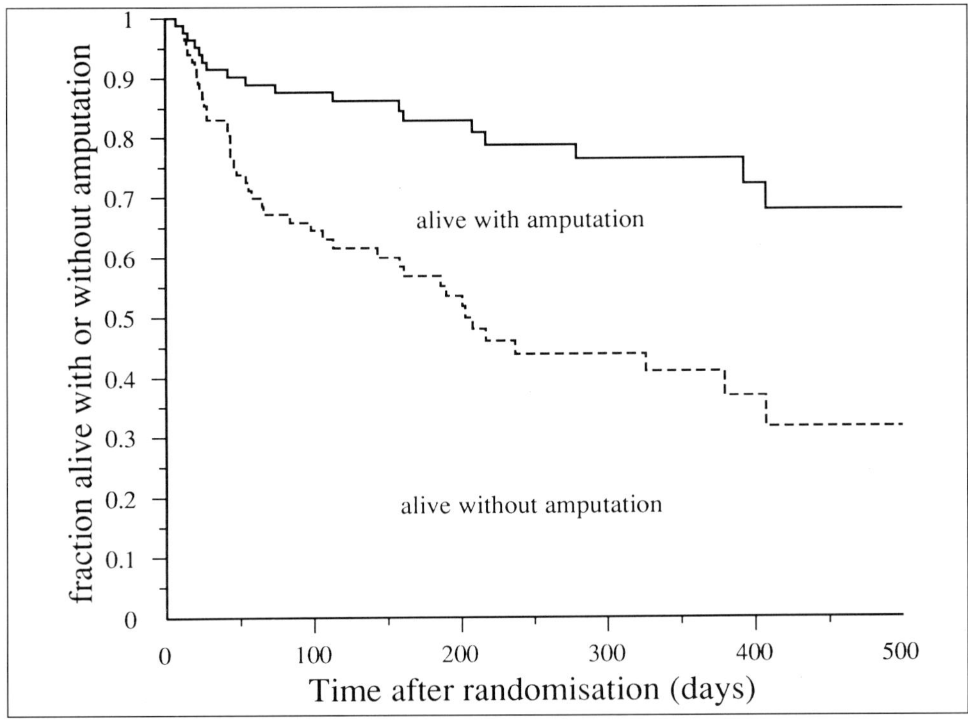

Fig. 5. Kaplan-Meier plot for the whole group of trial patients, showing the percentage alive (upper line) and the percentage alive without amputation (lower line)

people representing the general English population. General well-being of trial patients proves to be much worse than well-being of the general population. Compared to other severely ill patients (liver and heart transplantation candidates), quality of life is also less, pain being the predominant characteristic. The results have been summarized in Fig. 4.

Follow-up: By July 1993, median follow-up was 6.5 months. Eighteen patients died, 28 patients underwent major amputation (foot or higher level). The Kaplan-Meier plot is shown in Fig. 5. The lowest area indicates the proportion of patients alive without amputation. The area between the two curves indicates the proportion of patients alive with amputation. At 365 days, it can be read that 76% of the patients are still alive: 41% without amputation and 35% with an amputation. It can be concluded, that, as expected, the incidence of death and amputation is high in this group of patients. In statistical terms, this means that a notable outcome improvement from treatment, if present, should be detectable.

Summary

The ESES-trial is a randomized controlled clinical trial to evaluate the effects of epidural electrical spinal cord stimulation as compared to standard treatment in patients with critical limb ischemia. This pragmatic trial will be analyzed according to the intention-to-treat principle with patient survival, limb survival, quality of life and

181

cost-effectiveness, as primary outcome measures. From November 1991 until July 1993, 90 patients were enrolled. Considering the high incidence of deaths and amputations, 18 months of follow-up seems adequate. We hope to present the results of this study at the end of 1994.

References

1. Augustinsson L (1987) Epidural spinal electrical stimulation in peripheral vascular disease. PACE 10:205–206
2. Augustinsson L, Holm J, Carlsson CA, Jivegard L (1985) Epidural electrical stimulation in severe limb ischemia. Evidences of pain relief increased blood flow and a possible limb-saving effect. Ann Surg 202:104–111
3. Bracale GC, Selvetella L, Mirabile F (1989) Our experience with spinal cord stimulation (SCS) in peripheral vascular disease. PACE 12:695–697
4. Broseta J, Barbera J, Vera JA de, Barcia-Salorio JL, Garcia-March G, Gonzalez-Darder J, Rovaina F, Joanes V (1986) Spinal cord stimulation in peripheral arterial disease. J Neurosurg 64:71–80
5. Cook AW, Oygar A, Baggenstos P, Pacheco S, Kleriga E (1976) Vascular disease of extremities: Electric stimulation of spinal cord and posterior roots. NY State J of Med:366–368
6. Dormandy J, Mahir M, Ascady G, Balsano F, Leeuw P de, Blombery P (1989) Fate of the patient with chronic leg ischemia. J Cardiovasc Surg 30:50–57
7. Dormandy JA, Mahir MS (1986) The natural history of peripheral atheromatous disease of legs. In: Vascular surgery: Issues in current practice, Grune & Stratton, pp 3–17
8. Fiume D, Palombi M, Sciassa V, Tamorri M (1989) Spinal cord stimulation (SCS) in peripheral ischemic pain. PACE 12:698–704
9. Fowkes FGR (1988) Epidemiology of atherosclerotic arterial disease in the lower limbs. Eur J Vasc Surg 2:283–291
10. Jacobs MJHM, Jorning PJG, Beckers RCY, Ubbink DT, Kleef M van (1990) Foot salvage and improvement of microvascular blood flow as a result of epidural spinal cord electrical stimulation. J Vasc Surg 12(3):354–360
11. Jivegard L, Augustinsson L, Carlsson C, Holm J (1987) Long-term results by epidural spinal electrical stimulation (ESES) in patients with inoperable severe lower limb ischemia. Eur J Vasc Surg 1:345–349
12. Pocock SJ (1983) Blinding and Placebos in SJ Pocock (eds) clinical trials. John Wiley & Sons Ltd, pp 90–100
13. Sampere CT, Guasch JA, Paladino CM, Casalongue S, Elencwajg B (1989) Spinal cord stimulation for severely ischemic limbs. PACE 12:273–279
14. Thompson MM, Sayers RD, Varty K, Reid A, London NJM, Bell PRF (1993) Chronic critical leg ischemia must be redefined. Eur J Vasc Surg 7:420–426
15. Schwartz D, Lellouch J (1967) Explanatory and pragmatic attitudes in therapeutical trials. J Chron Dis 20:637–648
16. Tallis RC, Illis LS, Sedgwick EM, Hardwidge C, Garfield JS (1983) Spinal cord stimulation in peripheral vascular disease. J Neurology Neurosurgery and Psychiatry 46:478–484
17. Troidl H (1991) Quality of life: definition conceptualization and implications – a surgeon's view. Theor Surg 6:138–142
18. Zelen M (1974) The randomization and stratification of patients to clinical trials. J Chron Dis 27:365–375

Authors' address:

H. M. Klomp, M. D., G. H. J. J. Spincemaille, M. D.
Coordination Center ESES-trial
Dept. of General Surgery
Vascular Unit
University Hospital Rotterdam-Dijkzigt
Dr. Molewaterplein 40, NL-3015 GD Rotterdam, The Netherlands

182

Spinal cord stimulation in peripheral vascular disease treatment: Nine-year experience with 241 patients

F. Zucco*, B. Allaria*, M. Vaghi**, F. Rizzi*, W. Reina*, E. Boselli*, S. Brusa*, A. Tacconi**

*Anaesthesiological department, **Vascular department, Santa Corona Hospital, Garbagnate Milanese

Introduction

Spinal cord stimulation is still a controversial approach in the treatment of chronic pain, in the last 10 years it was extensively used in Europe to treat the symptoms of peripheral vascular disease.

The gate theory [18] represents a useful, rational foundation for the evaluation of experimental and clinical applications of spinal cord electroanalgesia. However, the precise mechanism of electro-mediated analgesia has still not been elucidated.

Currently the most widespread application of SCS in Europe is in the symptomatic treatment of peripheral obstructive and vasospastic vascular disease (PVD) (Table 1). The main objective of this article is to summarize the state of the art in the application of SCS to PVD.

Controlled instrumental techniques demonstrated that SCS increased peripheral blood flow [4, 10, 14, 19, 21] in addition to its well established analgesic properties, and this naturally extended the clinical use of SCS to treat PVD symptoms and signs (rest pain, claudication pain, ischemic ulcers). SCS application to arteriopathic patients was highly successful, not only in reducing pain, but the therapy is now also considered to be an indirect revascularization technique rather than being simply analgesic [22]. SCS capacity to increase residual blood flow reserve in peripheral ischemic areas, combined with its analgesic effect, makes it advantageous compared

Table 1. SCS in peripheral vascular disease

Author	No. of patients	Trial period days	N. stimulators implanted (NI)	Ratio NI/EI* %	Follow-up months
Tallis (1983)	9	10	4	44	6 – 26
Augustinsson (1985)	34	no	34	100	1 – 78
Broseta (1986)	41	yes (?)	37	90	2 – 48
Broggi (1987)	40	7 – 30	31	77	?
Bracale (1989)	27	5 – 14	25	92	?
Fiume (1989)	54	7 – 15	45	83	48
Franzetti (1989)	32	7 – 10	27	84	4 – 18
Galley (1990)	202	9	177	87	2 – 41
Izzo (1990)	12	14 – 28	3	25	?
Jacobs (1990)	20	3	18	90	3 – 36
Bunt (1991)	15	no	15	100	12
Zucco (1992)	139	21	84	60	24

*NI/EI: Neurostimulators implanted/Electrodes implanted

to other less expensive mainly pain-controlling therapeutic approaches (e.g., continuous epidural chemical neuromodulation with local anesthetics and/or opioids). To date, no studies have been published comparing SCS to pharmacological (e.g., i.v. prostacyclins) or indirect revascularization approaches (e.g., surgical or chemically induced lesions or anesthetic block of the sympathetic system), and only a few authors [1, 10, 22, 23] have evaluated the efficacy of SCS on previously sympathectomized arteriopathic patients. In no case were these results compared to non-sympathectomized controls. Furthermore, none of the study schemes have employed third party-independent evaluators.

The studies reporting on instrumental monitoring of SCS-induced modifications to peripheral blood flow are particularly interesting [4, 10, 14, 15, 19, 21]: it is on these works, performed on both animals and humans, that the clinical use of SCS on PVD is rationally based.

Our experience of SCS use in PVD

Over the period 1986 to 1993, we implanted 241 epidural, mostly unipolar electrodes for the treatment of various chronic pain syndromes. 218 of these patients were affected by ischemic pain secondary to lower limb arteriopathy of varying etiology and severity. None of these patients was suitable for other therapeutic approaches, for clinical or other reasons related to the type of arteriopathy. Patient selection was performed by a team consisting of vascular surgeons and anesthetists experienced in SCS and other analgesic techniques. The electrodes were always implanted by the same operator. The vascular results pertaining to the first 139 patients of this series are presented here (Table 2 and 3). Dedicated software was used to analyze these results and manage the data stored in three different data bases: 1) patient history and temporary stimulation data, 2) permanent neurostimulator follow-up, 3) pain control analysis.

Confining ourselves to vascular conditions, we compared the number of patients with a positive response to SCS to the non-responder group, we included in the latter category patients previously implanted with an epidural electrode and who subsequently underwent thigh or leg amputation, or emergency revascularization surgery.

A two-step implantation schedule is now used by almost all operators: after epidural electrode implantation a period of assessment follows which, depending on the center, may last from 2 days to 4 weeks (Table 1) and is variously referred to as the temporary, test, testing or external period. At the end of this period a decision is made to implant a permanent neurostimulator or remove the electrode, depending on the clinical response. A precise and quantitative evaluation of SCS-mediated analgesia is required to identify responders and hence decide whether to implant a

Table 2. SCS in 139 PVD patients: Etiology

Pathology	No. of patients
1) Atherosclerosis	93
2) Mixed (atherosclerosis plus diabetes)	39
3) Diabetic microangiopathy	6
4) Sclerodermic Raynaud	1

184

Table 3. SCS clinical results in 139 PVD patients

Fontaine class	No. of patients	% N.S./E.I.	% of responders		
			6 months	12 months	24 months
2 B	24	96	96 (22)	89 (15)	89 (8)
3	35	57	54 (18)	47 (13)	41 (7)
4 A	60	53	37 (19)	37 (18)	29 (7)
4 B	20	45	15 (3)	15 (3)	7 (1)
Total	139	60			

2 B: Claudication free interval less than 50 meters
3:   Rest pain without ischemic cutaneous lesions (i.c.l.)
4 A: Rest pain with nongangrenous i.c.l.
4 B: Rest pain with gangrenous i.c.l.
Numbers in brackets indicate the number of patients evaluated at each specific follow-up time

neurostimulator (Table 4). To achieve this, we employed a complex system based on three different pain scales (semantic, analogue, numerical) as well as on the score of a specifically prepared drug consumption scale. Each scale had a 0 to 10 range. In all cases clinical evaluations were performed at fixed times: basal (2–3 days before electrode implantation), once a week during the test period, and at the end of the external stimulation period (after a minimum of three weeks trial at our center). In the patients who received a permanent neurostimulator implant, outcome was evaluated at 1, 3, 6, and 12 months and, subsequently, yearly. In all 241 cases the follow-up included evaluation of technical problems and complications.

Since 1989, we have used short-term prophylaxis with cefazoline, 1 g i.v. 30 min before the surgical procedure.

Results

The results are shown in Tables 1 and 3. The ratio of number of (permanent) neurostimulators implanted (NS) to number of electrodes originally implanted (EI) is regarded by many authors as an indirect index of the short-term clinical effectiveness of SCS. As Table 1 shows, our NS/EI index (60%) is among the lowest, only Izzo [13] and Tallis [21] report lower ratios (25% and 44%, respectively). Both of these studies involved very small series of patients (12 and 9, respectively). Our low NS/EI index is probably due to our more restricted definition of responder (Table 4), rather than to technical differences between the studies.

It is also important to note that the percentages of responders at different follow-up times in our study were calculated with reference to the total number of electrode

Table 4. SCS in 139 PVD patients: Criteria for evaluation of SCS responders

Class 2 B: Walking free interval allows independent life
Class 3 :   more than 50% reduction in rest pain
Class 4 :   more than 50% reduction in rest pain
             evidence of ulcer healing in progress or delimitation of gangrenous area

implantations originally carried out. The technical problems and complications we observed are summarized in Tables 5a, b, and c.

Table 5a. SCS in 241 patients: Complications and problems

Period	Pathology	N. of pts.	%
Intra-operative	Cardiac block (reversible)	1	0.2
	Symptomatic bradycardia	5	1.1
	Dural puncture	7*	2.5
Post-operative (6 h)	Cardio/respiratory failure (not reversible: exitus)	1	0.2
	Symptomatic bradycardia	2	0.4
	Post. superficial hematoma	1	0.2
	Ant. superficial hematoma (neurostimulator pocket)	3**	0.6
Post-operative (1 w)	Cardiac failure (not reversible: exitus)	1	0.2
	Ictus cerebri (not reversible: exitus)	1	0.2
	Probable meningitus (not reversible: exitus)	1*	0.4
	Persistent severe headache (lasting 1 week)	2*	0.7

* % calculated from the total number of electrode implantations
** % calculated from the number of neurostimulators implanted

Table 5b. SCS in 241 patients: Complications and problems

Pathology	No. of patients	%
Superficial infections		
within 15 days after surgery	6*	1.3
after the 15-day post-operative period	3*	0.7
before 1989	8**	4.2
after 1989 (cefazoline 1 g i.v. in short-term prophylaxis)	1***	0.4

* % calculated from the total of electrode (EL) and neurostimulator (NE) implantations
** % calculated from the total of EL and NE before 1989
*** % calculated from the total of EL and NE after 1989

Table 5c. SCS in 241 patients: Electrode displacements

Type of displacement	No. of patients	%
Cephalad migration	3	1.1
Caudal migration out of epidural space	13	5.3
Caudal migration into the epidural space	10	3.8
Total	26	9.8
Electrode reimplant	11	5.0
Patients who refused reimplant	2	0.8

Discussion

From an analysis of the studies published to date and from our experience, it is possible to draw a number of conclusions concerning the utility of and indications for SCS:

1) In arteriopathic patients SCS can be useful if pharmacological or surgical treatments are not possible or prove to be ineffective. Some authors designate absolute and relative indications for SCS in PVD (Table 6).
2) Contrary to the recommendations of the early reports [1, 10, 22], in our opinion SCS should not be used to treat patients affected by extensive gangrenous lesions of the foot (in Europe, these patients are classified in Fontaine's fourth B stage). The best treatment for these patients is pain control associated with continuous care of the lesions. From our experience, in the presence of severe nociceptive somatic pain the analgesia associated with SCS is less effective than that obtained with epidural anesthetics with or without opiates.

    Concerning patients affected by only claudication ischemic pain, we feel that electrode implantation is indicated if the pain-free walking interval (PFWI) is less than 50 meters (Fontaine's second B stage patients) and if other therapeutic options have definitely been excluded.
3) The presence of diabetes does not represent a contraindication to the use of SCS.
4) At present, it is not clear if intact sympathetic function is a necessary condition for SCS effectiveness in peripheral vascular disease [1, 4, 5, 10, 13, 17]. It is necessary to carry out controlled clinical studies to compare the efficacy of SCS with that of sympathetic neuromodulative or neurolesive approaches.

    In patients affected by ischemic pain at rest without lesions (Fontaine's third stage) or by small peripheral ischemic ulcers (Fontaine's fourth A stage), the indications for SCS and sympathetic intervention (ablative or blocking) may overlap.
5) In arteriopathy, the aim of SCS is not only to achieve effective analgesia (which might be obtained by other less expensive techniques), but also to effect trophic-functional recovery of the body segment affected by an advanced ischemic process.
6) It is of utmost importance that the external testing period following electrode implantation be at least 2–3 weeks: this is the minimum time necessary to check the patients and their clinical response adequately, so that the number of neuro-stimulator implantations in so-called false responders is kept to a minimum. Such an approach is important for limiting costs.

Table 6. Peripheral vascular disease: Indications for spinal cord stimulation

Absolute:	Patients in whom angiography indicates the impossibility of direct vascularization a) Fontaine's 2ndB, 3rd and 4thA stages b) Not previously sympathectomized
Relative:	Patients in whom angiography indicates technical possibility of revascularisation but with elevated risks for surgery: a) anesthesiological general risks b) risk of surgical inefficacy

7) During the testing period it is necessary that, in addition to pain control, the effect on peripheral blood flow is carefully assessed. This assessment should include determination of the pain-free walking interval under standard conditions (treadmill), confirmation of ulcer healing (by photographs, surface measurements, etc.) and verification of improved blood flow. The most useful instrumental techniques for peripheral vascular screening during SCS are plethysmography and transcutaneous PO_2 ($TCPO_2$).

8) Further studies are required to define the optimum characteristics regarding the intensity and the temporal pattern of the stimulation.

9) In spite of the fact that the electrode is implanted percutaneously under local anesthesia, the SCS technique is not totally risk free, and its use should be limited to hospitals employing specially trained medical and nursing staff.

References

1. Augustinsson LE, Holm J, Carlsson AC, Jivegard L (1985) Epidural electrical stimulation in severe limb ischemia. Evidence of pain relief, increased blood flow and a possible limb-saving effect. Annals of Surgery 202:104–111
2. Bracale GC, Selvetella L, Mirabile F (1989) Our experience with spinal cord stimulation in peripheral vascular disease. Pace 12:695–697
3. Broggi G, Servello D, Franzini A (1987) Spinal cord stimulation for treatment of peripheral vascular disease. Appl Neurophysiol 50:439–441
4. Broseta J, Barbera J, De Vera JA, et al. (1986) Spinal cord stimulation in peripheral arterial disorders. Co-operative study. J Neurosurg 64:71–80
5. Bunt TJ (1991) Letters to editors. J Vasc Surg 14:829
6. Cook AW, Oygar A, Baggenstos P, Pacheco S, Kleriga S (1978) Vascular disease of extremities: electrical stimulation of spinal cord and posterior roots. NY St J Med 76:366–368
7. Dooley D, Pasproak M (1976) Modification of blood flow to the extremities by electrical stimulation of the nervous system. South Med J 69:1309–1311
8. Fiume D (1983) Spinal cord stimulation in peripheral vascular pain. Appl Neurophysiol 39:534–546
9. Franzetti L, De Nale A, Bossi A (1989) Epidural spinal electrostimulatory system (ESES) in the management of diabetic foot and peripheral artheriopathies. Pace 1 12:705–708
10. Galley D, Elharrar C, Schefer J, Jeangeorges B, Serena G (1989) Neurostimulation et pathologie vasculaire: interet therapeutique. A propos de 49 patients. Coeur 20:35–44
11. Graber JN, Lifson A (1987) The use of spinal cord stimulation for severe limb-threatening ischemia: a preliminary report. Ann Vasc Surg 1:578–582
12. Hilton SM, Marshall JM (1980) Dorsal root vasodilatation in cat skeletal muscle. J Physiol (London) 299:277–288
13. Izzo V, Mariconti P, Tiengo M (1990) Absence of sympathetic activity and spinal cord stimulation in advanced stages of arteriosclerosis obliterans. Pain Clinic 3:169–172
14. Jacobs MJ, Jorning PJG, Beckers RCY (1990) Foot salvage and improvement of microvascular blood flow as a result of epidural spinal cord stimulation. J Vasc Surg 12:354–360
15. Linderoth B, Fedorcsack I, Meyerson BA (1991) Peripheral vasodilatation after spinal cord stimulation: animal studies of putative effector mechanism. Neurosurg 1 28:187–195
16. Linderoth B, Gunasekera L, Meyerson BA (1991) Effects of sympathectomy on skin and muscle microcirculation during dorsal column stimulation in men. Neurosurg 29:874–879
17. Linderoth B, Gazelis B, Frank J, Brodin E (1992) Dorsal column stimulation induces release of serotonin and substance P in the cat dorsal horn. Neurosurg 31:289–297
18. Melzack R, Wall PD (1965) Pain mechanism: a new theory. Science 150:971–979

19. Sciacca V, Mingoli A, Di Marzo L, Maggiore C, Fiume D, Cavallaro A (1989) Predictive value of transcutaneous oxygen tension measurement in the indication for spinal cord stimulation in patients with peripheral vascular disease: preliminary results. Vasc Surg 23, 2:128–132
20. Sciacca V, Mingoli A, Maggiore C (1991) Laser Doppler flowmetry and transcutaneous oxygen tension with severe arterial insufficiency treated by epidural spinal cord stimulation. Vasc Surg 25, 3:165–170
21. Tallis RC, Illis LS, Sedgwick EM, Hardwidge C, Garfield JS (1983) Spinal cord stimulation in peripheral vascular disease. J Neurol Neurosurg Psych 46:478–484
22. Zucco F, Allaria B, Tacconi A (1988) Unipolar spinal cord stimulation in lower limb vascular disease: causal or symptomatic therapy? A review of 107 cases. XXVI World Cong Int Cong Surgeons abs (Monduzzi ed), 532
23. Zucco F, Allaria B, Rizzi F (1992) Pain control in PVD: 138 patients with epidural electrical stimulation. 5th Int Congress The pain clinic, abs Jerusalem, 37

Authors' address:

Zucco F., M.D.
Anaesthesiological Department
Santa Corona Hospital
Garbagnate Milanese
I-Milano
Italy

Spinal cord stimulation – Multicentral spanish study

E. Viver, S. Llagostera, J. R. Escudero, L. Olba, C. García

Vascular Surgery Dpt., Hospital de Sant Pau – Barcelona, Spain

Introduction

The stimulation of the medulla's rear cords is being used at present for several treatments:
1) to fight against the tremor shown by patients with Parkinson disease;
2) for the pain caused by an lasting angor;
3) for the peripheral vascular disease of lower extremities of an atheromatous origin in which there are not surgical possibilities.

The basis of the medullar application is founded on some experimental works published in the years 1973 and 1974 by Cook and Dooley [2], and on the multicenter studies at European level made in 1986 and 1990. In Spain, the first to apply this method were Dr. Azcona and colleagues of the Faculty of Medicine of Zaragoza and Dr. Herreros of the Faculty of Medicine of Navarra.

The works of Jacobs [3] (1988), Meglio [4] (1981) and Augustinnson [1] (1989), measuring the increase of cutaneous blood flow, helped the authors to arrive at the following conclusions.
1) A diminution of the ischemic pains of about 75 – 80%;
2) an increase of the walking distance;
3) an improvement in the evolution of the ischemic trophic injuries;
4) a diminution in the amputation rate.

AIM and design

After a preliminary phase, during which some neuro-stimulators in experimental phase were implanted in several hospitals in Spain, we arrived at a general assent about the convenience and usefulness of making a national multicenter study in Spain, to evaluate the effectiveness of this treatment on patients with vascular pathology who are not candidates for reconstructive arterial surgery.

To this aim a committee of specialists prepared a program with standards of inclusion and exclusion and for follow-up of the patient's during 18 months.

The protocol's aim is addressed to three correlated directions:

1) improvement or disappearance of the rest pain;
2) heating of the trophic injuries;
3) decrease of the amputation rate.

Type of test

This is a clinical test, prospective, with centralized aleatory selection, multicenter with a common protocol, and final evaluation by a committee.

In the beginning the number of patients to be observed is 300 and the period of follow-up is 18 months. It is considered a success the conservation of the extremity in a functional state and without rest pain is considered successful and is considered a failure amputation.

Standards of inclusion

Patients affected by peripheral arteriopathy of the lower extremities with rest pain, superficial ulcers, minimal ischemic injuries and without possibilities of direct arterial surgery. The angiography had to have, at maximum, conducted no move than two months previously.

Standards of exclusion

Buerguers disease
Raynauds disease
Coagulation disorders
Wet gangrene
Deep ulcers
Cutaneous necrotic injuries
Psychic-social problems of the patient
Refusal to sign the consent.

Once the consent signature was obtained, the patients were aleatorially selected at each center to be in one of the two groups:
1) Abstention — Rheologic treatment;
2) Neuro-stimulator (SCS).

In the first group the abstention refers to not applying the SCS; another kind of treatment can be recommended (except surgery) as, for instance, prostaglandin, rheologic, vasodilators; the type and class of product used and the obtained result is them recorded.

The SCS is appraised according to pre-established techniques and an external generator is used; after 2 to 5 days, once its efficay is verified, the definitive one is installed.

The patients are examined after 1, 3, 6, 12 and 18 months.

The basic differences between the Spanish Protocol and the European Protocol lay in two points: The implantation of an external neuro-stimulator, and the non inclusion of patients already showing ischemic injuries in the foot.

The first point, otherwise to place an external neurostimulator, is based on economic reasons. The price of a neurostimulator, in Spain, is very high, and we believe that the economics of our nation justifies the prevention of certain expenses that, in some cases, may be useless. Nevertheless, when the indications become more previse and the successes rates higher than the failures, we may modify this concept, but always with an experience that will guarantee a minimal amount of treatment mistakes.

Concerning the point of applying a neuro-stimulator in the presence of injuries, trophic or not, in reality it is very difficult to classify these injuries. There is a difference between an interdigital ulcer and an ulcer in the metatarsus phalanxic of the first finger with exposed tendon; this also applies to the deepness and extension of ulcer. If we could manage to obtain a classification allowing us an identification of the injury, we could arrive at some conclusions that would allow us, after some experience, to know in which types of injuries we could apply, with guarantees of success, the neuro-stimulator, and which types of injuries are prone to an amputation.

We propose the following classification:

1) superficial injury affecting the skin and the subcutaneous cellular tissue, of an extension up to 2 cm;
2) interdigital ulcerative injury affecting the bone that can necessitate amputation of the finger;
3) ulcer with exposition of the tendons;
4) ulcer with exposition of the bone (metatarsus, malleolus);
5) manifold injuries in different areas of the foot.

In the beginning, and a priori, only in the two first cases is the neuro-stimulator appropriate.

Conclusions

The treatment with neuron-stimulator of the patients with peripheral vascular pathology, in whom all surgical possibilities have been exhausted, is being accepted at present as an alternative, as are pharmacological and rheological treatments.

Our experience with this treatment is dictating its adaptation. In Spain, there are at present a few centers in which neuro-stimulators have been implanted in sufficient numbers to allow us to draw conclusions and, what is more important, to obtain clinical indications. At the present time (October 1993), a multicenter study that will include 300 patients and a follow-up of 18 months is in the process of being initiated.

We are convinced that at the end of that study the implantation indications of the neuron-stimulator will be certain.

References

1. Augustinnson LE (1985) Epidural electrical stimulation in severe limb ischemia: evidence of pain relief, increased blood flow and a possible limb-saving effect. Ann Surg 202:104–111
2. Dooley DM, Kasprak M (1973) Modification of blood flow to the extremities by electrical stimulation of the nervous system. South Med J 69:1309–1311
3. Jacobs JH MJ et al (1988) Epidural spinal cord stimulation improves microvascular blood flow in severe limb ischemia. Ann Surg 207:179–183
4. Meglio M et al (1981) Pain control and improvement of peripheral blood flow following epidural spinal cord stimulation. J Neurosurg 54:821–823

Authors' address:

Dr. E. Viver Mauresa
Hospital de La Santa Cren/Sant Pan
Hospital Universitari de La Facultat de Medicina de
La Universitat Autonoma de Barcelona
Sant Antoni M. Claret, 167
08025 Barcelona
Spain

Spinal cord stimulation (SCS) in patients with inoperable severe lower limb ischemia.
A prospective randomized controlled study of tissue loss and limb salvage

L. E. H. Jivegård, L.-E. Augustinsson[2], J. Holm, B. Risberg[1], P. Örtenwall[1]

Departments of Surgery, Sahlgrenska and [1]Östra Hospitals and
[2]Department of Neurosurgery, Sahlgrenska Hospital, Göteborg, Sweden

Spinal cord stimulation (SCS) reduces pain as well as improves microcirculatory parameters in ischemic limbs and it has been suggested that SCS may save limbs in patients with inoperable arterial occlusions. No randomized controlled study has been published, however.

In this study, performed in two vascular centers, atherosclerotic (n = 41) and diabetic (n = 10) patients having chronic leg ischemia with rest pain and/or ischemic ulcerations due to inoperable arterial occlusions were randomized to SCS and analgesic treatment (n = 25) or analgesic and conservative treatment (controls, n = 26). The patients were followed regarding macrocirculatory parameters, pain relief, limb salvage, and tissue loss (classified as none or only forefoot amputation/amputation below knee/above knee/bilateral amputation) for at least 18 months.

Macrocirculatory parameters were not different in the two groups during follow-up. Long-term pain relief was significant only in the SCS group. Limb salvage rates in the SCS and control groups were 62% and 45% (n.s.) at 18 months, while tissue loss was significantly smaller at 24 months in the SCS group. In normotensive patients, the amputation rate was lower (p < 0.05) in the SCS vs the control group at 18 months.

It is concluded that SCS may reduce tissue loss in patients with severe inoperable leg ischemia and is likely to improve long-term limb salvage in subgroups of such patients. The present results suggest that patients who do not have established arterial hypertension constitute a subgroup of particular interest in future studies of limb salvage in response to SCS.

Authors' address:

Jivegård L. MD
Dept. of Surgery
University of Göteborg
Sahlgrenska Hospital
S-41345 Göteborg
Sweden

Spinal cord stimulation for ischemic rest pain.
The Belgian randomized study

R. Suy[1], J. Gybels[1], H. Van Damme[2], D. Martin[2], R. van Maele[3],
C. Delaporte[3]

[1]K.U. Leuven, [2]C.H.U. Liège, [3]U.I. Antwerpen, Belgium

A prospective randomized study was performed at three Belgium university hospitals
to evaluate the possible benefit of spinal cord stimulation (SCS) on severe limb
ischemia. The study started in November 1989 and the last patient was randomised
on March 1992. The final evaluation was done in August 1993.

The aim of the study was to evaluate:

1) the analgesic effect of SCS on ischemic pain;
2) the healing effect of SCS on ischemic ulcers;
3) the limb salvage effect of SCS.

The inclusion criteria were:

1) chronic ischemic rest pain related to peripheral vascular occlusive disease, either
   due to arteriosclerosis (ASD) or to arteritis (Buerger's disease);
2) the presence of severe arteriopathy, unsuitable for vascular reconstruction,
   angioplasty or thrombolysis. Appropriate arteriographies, performed shortly before randomization, were evaluated by an experienced vascular surgeon.
3) limitation of existing trophic lesions to superficial ulcers without involvement of
   tendons or bone, or to dry or wet gangrene of a toe.

The clinical material

Thirty-eight patients were randomized, 20 for implantation of an SCS device (called
the "Implant group") and 18 for further conservative treatment (called the "Control
group"). Smokers were advised to stop smoking completely and all patients received
an optimal medical treatment consisting of appropriate antiaggregation therapy,
rheological medication and analgesic therapy, including toe amputation if necessary.
Thirty of the 38 patients were on narcotic analgesic treatment at the time of randomization.

Patient demographic data are listed in Table 1. There were no statistically significant differences in data between the two groups. There was a non-significant trend
in smoking habits between the two groups: nine of the 20 patients of the Implant
group continued to smoke or resumed smoking during the follow-up period, versus
13 of the 18 patients in the Control group (p = 0.12). A more detailed characteriza-
tion of symptoms than in the Fontaine classification was used since we believe that
a cold, cyanotic, livid forefoot or gangrene of a toe have a less favourable prognosis
than ischemia without these characteristics, such as uncomplicated rest pain or rest
pain with ulcers.

Table 1. Patient demographics

	SCS (n = 20)	Control (n = 18)
Male/female ratio	15/5	15/3
Age (years)		
mean ASD	66 ± 11	65 ± 9
Buerger's	36 ± 10	46 ± 9
range	26 – 80	36 – 80
Etiology		
Arteriosclerosis (ASD)	16	11
Arteritis (Buerger's disease)	4	7
Localization of lesions		
foot arteries	3	0
crural arteries	5	9
femoropopliteal arteries	12	8
external iliac artery + femoropopliteal arteries	0	1
Symptomatology		
uncomplicated rest pain	5	4
rest pain and ulcers	6	7
livid cyanotic forefoot	3	2
dry toe gangrene	4	4
wet gangrene	2	1
Previous vascular operations		
sympathectomy	8	13
vascular reconstruction	10	11
number of operations	26	23
Risk factors for occlusive disease		
diabetes mellitus		
type I	3	1
type II	3	1
nicotine usage		
non-smoker	3	0
stopped months before	2	5
stopped at entry of the study	6	0
stopped but resumed	1	3
continued smoking	8	10

Hardware, and Implant

All patients had Medtronic model 3587A (Resume) leads implanted in the epidural space at D9 – 11 through laminectomy by a neurosurgeon. In the same procedure (without trial screening) 11 patients received a bipolar implanted pulse generator (IPG) model 7420 and nine patients received a programmable IPG, model 7424.

There were three complications of the SCS implantation. One early device infection led to complete device removal and reimplantation of a new device at a higher level. There was also one early disconnection and one late broken wire in other patients 2 years after implantation, both necessitating surgical correction.

Study, design

At the moment of randomization all patients had an evaluation of pain with a visual analogue scale (VAS) from 1 to 10, a microcirculation test (TcPO2 measurement at the middle of the forefoot) and a macrocirculation test (Doppler test for ankle/brachial pressure index). It was planned to repeat these tests a 1 week, 3, 6 and 12 months and later on a yearly basis. However, a lot of these data are missing since many of the patients, especially those of the control group, would not come back on regular scheduled times.

The endpoints of the study were death without previous amputation, or a major amputation. A transmetatarsal amputation was considered as major since this amputation was only performed in patients with normal femoropopliteal and proximal crural arteries. Their pathology was mainly localized in the pedalarteries and, therefore, a loss of the forefoot was considered as a major amputation.

Results (Table 2)

The mean follow-up time was 20 ± 15 months. Eight patients (four of the implant and four of the control group) died since the start of the study. The causes of death were mesenteric infarction (1), cancer (2), terminal cardiac disease (2), stroke (1), cachexia related to refusal of amputation of the contralateral limb (1) and unknown (1).

Four patients (one in the Implant group and three in the Control group) had a late vascular event. Surgical repair (one embolectomy and one angioplasty) reversed two patients to their clinical state before the incident. In two patients of the control group a below-knee amputation was performed.

1. Amputation rate

A previously scheduled *toe* amputation was performed in seven patients. Three of these patients were pain-free after amputation. Three patients underwent later additional toe amputations and in one patient a below-knee amputation had to be performed 8 months later.

A *major* amputation was necessary in 15 patients (Fig. 1). Six of the 20 patients of the Implant group underwent a major amputation versus nine of the 18 of the

Table 2. Clinical results

		SCS (n = 20)	Control (n = 18)
a.	Excellent	9	1
b.	Good	5	4
c.	Unchanged	0	4
d.	Deterioration (major amputation)	6	9
	forefoot amputation	1	2
	below knee amputation	4	5
	above knee amputation	1	2

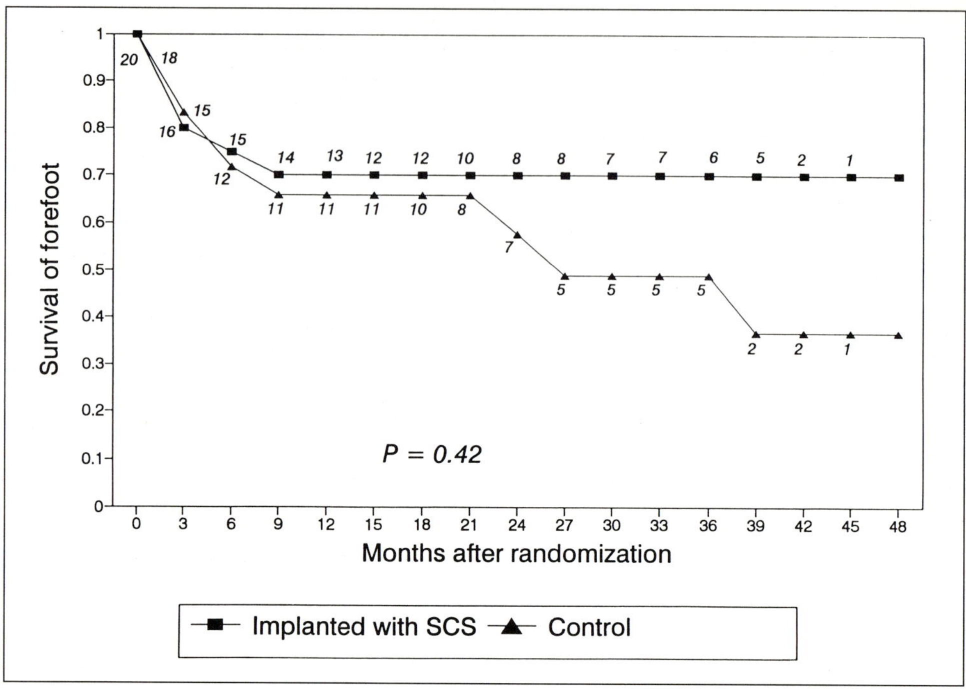

Fig. 1. Forefoot survival lifetable curve, avoidance of a transmetatarsal or below-knee or above-knee amputation. p-value is from a chi-square log rank test. The numbers along the curves are the patients entering each interval

control group. Ten amputations had to be performed within 6 months after randomization. The survival curves without a major amputation look very similar up to 21 months. There were three additional late amputations in the control group: two of these patients had a late vascular incident, confirmed by arteriography and in both patients a below-knee amputation was necessary. In part, due to low patient enrolement, the curves in Fig. 1 are not significantly different (p = 0.42).

2. Clinical result

An evaluation was made at 12 and 24 months. The clinical result of the treatment, either with or without SCS implant, is classified as follows:

Class 1 *Excellent result:* Complete relief of ischemic rest pain, no limitation of walking distance for daily activities, normal social life, healing of ulcers (if present) or demarcation of gangrene with subsequent healing.

Class 2 *Good result:* Complete relief of rest pain with, however, still some restrictions such as toe-amputation, imcomplete healing of a painless ulcer or (and) incapacitating claudication.

Class 3 *Unchanged:* still analgesic drugs for rest pain, no cure of painful ulcers. Two patients in this class died without major amputations.

Class 4 *Deterioration* leading to major amputation (n = 15).

200

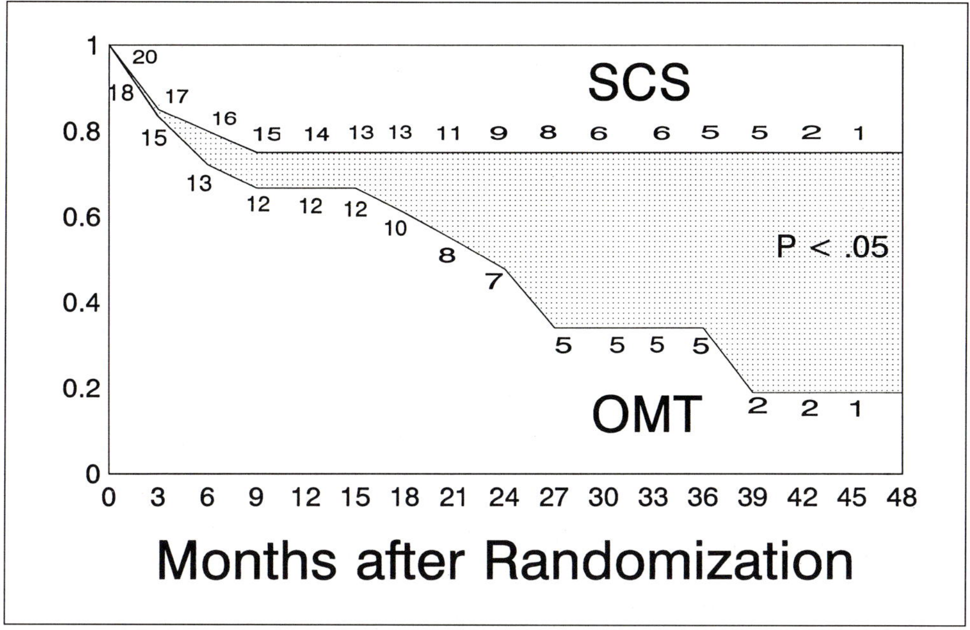

Fig. 2. Clinical success lifetable analysis. Outcome class 1 or class 2

Class 1 and 2 outcomes are considered to be clinically successful. From a clinical point of view, patients with an SCS implant did better than patients of the control group (Fig. 2), and the curves are statistically different (log rank test, p < 0.05).

Nine months after randomization, 15 of the 20 patients (75%) of the implant group belonged to class 1 or 2 versus 12 of the 18 patients (67%) of the control group.

Only 26 patients have a longer follow-up since two non-amputated patients died and 10 patients underwent a major amputation. At 12 months 13 of the 14 (93%) patients of the implant group belong to classes 1 or 2 versus eight of the 12 (67%) patients of the control group. One patient in each group underwent a major amputation between 6 and 12 months.

Seventeen patients have a follow-up longer than 12 months. At 24 months all eight patients of the implant group belong to classes 1 or 2 versus five of the nine (56%) patients of the control group. Three more patients of the control group were amputated by 24 months or later. Two of these late amputations were related to vascular events.

Risk Factors

A univariate analysis was made to determine the influence of several factors on the final outcome. Age, sex, presence of either type of diabetes and localization of the arterial pathology had no significant influence on outcome. Determining were, according to this univariate analysis, the etiology of the disease (ASD versus Buerger's disease), previous vascular surgery and especially smoking habits.

– The benefit of an SCS implant was most evident in patients with *arteriosclerotic disease*. Eleven of the 16 patients (68%) with implants went to classes 1 or 2 versus only two of 11 (18%) in the control group (p = 0.018).

– Twenty-one patients had previous *vascular surgery*. Fourty-nine reconstructions were performed in these 21 patients. Three grafts (one aortofemoral bypass and two femoropopliteal grafts) were still patent at the moment of randomization. Patients with a previous vascular operation did better with implant (six out of 10 successful versus only one of 11 patients in the control group) (p = 0.024).

– Patients who continued to *smoke* or who resumed smoking after the start of the study have a poor prognosis, independent of the type of treatment. Sixteen of the 38 patients never smoked or stopped smoking before randomization. Twelve of these 16 patients (75%) went to classes 1 or 2 (excellent or good results). On the other hand, 22 patients continued to smoke or resumed smoking. Only eight of these (36%) went to classes 1 or 2 at the end of the study (p = 0.025). The success rate of those who continued smoking was 5/9 for the implanted group and only 3/13 for the control group (p = 0.19).

– In patients without hyper*tension* the implanted group had a success rate of 11/14 versus 4/14 for the control group (p = 0.021). On the contrary, patients with hypertension had the same outcome regardless of the treatment.

– Patients with *umcomplicated rest pain or rest pain with superficial ulcerations* benefit from stimulation: success rate for the Implanted group was 10/11 versus 4/11 for the control group (p = 0.024). For more advanced situations (*livid food, gangrene*) no differential benefit was observed.

Conclusion

This randomized study evaluated both amputation rate and clinical outcome. No significant difference between either group was observed considering transmetatarsal amputation as major.

The clinical success however is also related to pain relief, ability to walk and quality of life. A clear benefit in favor of the implant group appeared. The size of the study however limits the ability to make strong conclusions. Several risk factors appeared to have significant correlations to outcome. A differential benefit of SCS versus conservative treatment was observed in normotensive patients with arteriosclerosis, especially after previous vascular procedures. Continuous smoking is without any doubt a bad prognostic factor.

The initial stage of the disease was found to be very important. Livid forefoot or gangrene may be a too advanced situation to have any benefit of an SCS implant.

Authors'address:

Prof. Dr. R. Suy
U.Z. Gasthuisberg
Dept. of Vascular Surgery
Herestraat 49
B-3000 Leuven
Belgium